Narrative-Based Practice in Health and Social Care

Narrative-Based Practice in Health and Social Care outlines a vision of how witnessing narratives, paying attention to them, and developing an ability to question them creatively, can make the person's emerging story the central focus of health and social care, and of healing.

This text gives an account of the practical application of ideas and skills from contemporary narrative studies to health and social care. Promoting narrative-based practice in everyday encounters with patients and clients, and in supervision, teaching, teamwork and management, it presents "Conversations Inviting Change," an established narrative-based model of interactional skills.

Underpinned by an account of theory from narrative studies and related fields, including communication theory and systems thinking, it is written for students and practitioners across a broad range of professions in primary and secondary health care and social care.

More information about "Conversations Inviting Change" is available at www. conversationsinvitingchange.com. This website includes podcasts, presentations and further teaching material as well as details of forthcoming courses, and is continually updated with information about the approach described in this book.

John Launer is Associate Dean at Health Education England, an Honorary Consultant at the Tavistock and Portman NHS Foundation Trust, and Associate Editor of the *Postgraduate Medical Journal*.

"Reading John Launer's *Narrative-Based Practice in Health and Social Care: Conversations Inviting Change* gave me a powerful surge of hope. John finds words to express our deepest thoughts and visions for a truly respectful and effective health care. His transparent prose brings his reader to experience the clarity and value of narrative practice. Reading John Launer, awakened by his purity of thought, falling under the spell of his idealism, charged by his optimism, I feel myself in the presence of those giants of vision and faithful representers of 'the other.' We all gather, with John as host, in the clearing of a narrative path toward wholeness. If you care for the sick, read this book."

– **Professor Rita Charon, Columbia University, USA**

"This book guides us through the rapids and challenges of how to conduct conversations that lead to meaningful change. John Launer articulates with wonderful simplicity the subtleties of a narrative-based approach which enables people in difficult situations to negotiate and realise new ways of going forward. Given the ubiquity of calls for change and innovation, this book must be everyone's first port of call to make sure their plans and initiatives benefit from Launer's transformational approach to narrative communication."

– **Professor Rick Iedema, King's College London, UK**

"How can practitioners and patients become more receptive and responsive to each other? Launer's book addresses this question, and resonates with today's policy preoccupations; the need to develop relationships between practitioners working with the same patients in the same teams to improve collaborative practice. Narrative-based practice has yet to receive the attention in interprofessional education that it merits. 'Conversations Inviting Change' offers a remedy for this that I shall certainly keep to hand."

– **Hugh Barr, President, the Centre for the Advancement of Interprofessional Education, UK**

Narrative-Based Practice in Health and Social Care

Conversations Inviting Change

Second edition

John Launer

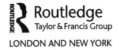

Routledge
Taylor & Francis Group

LONDON AND NEW YORK

Second edition published 2018
by Routledge
2 Park Square, Milton Park, Abingdon, Oxon, OX14 4RN

and by Routledge
711 Third Avenue, New York, NY 10017

Routledge is an imprint of the Taylor & Francis Group, an informa business

First edition published by CRC Press 2002

British Library Cataloguing-in-Publication Data
A catalogue record for this book is available from the British Library

Library of Congress Cataloging-in-Publication Data
Names: Launer, John, author.
Title: Narrative-based practice in health and social care / John Launer.
Other titles: Narrative-based primary care
Description: Second edition. | Abingdon, Oxon ; New York, NY :
    Routledge, 2018. | Preceded by Narrative-based primary care / John
    Launer. c2002. | Includes bibliographical references and index.
Identifiers: LCCN 2017047071| ISBN 9781138714373 (hardback) | ISBN
    9781138714359 (pbk.) | ISBN 9781315231129 (ebook)
Subjects: | MESH: Delivery of Health Care | Narration | Communication |
    Physician-Patient Relations
Classification: LCC RA418 | NLM W 84.1 | DDC 362.1—dc23
LC record available at https://lccn.loc.gov/2017047071

ISBN: 978-1-138-71437-3 (hbk)
ISBN: 978-1-138-71435-9 (pbk)
ISBN: 978-1-315-23112-9 (ebk)

Typeset in Sabon
by Swales & Willis Ltd, Exeter, Devon, UK
Printed and bound by CPI Group (UK) Ltd, Croydon CR0 4YY

For Lee, for Ruth, for David

Contents

Acknowledgements

The ideas in the book originated with the primary care course that ran at the Tavistock Clinic over many years. Apart from Caroline Lindsey and myself as organising tutors, the teaching staff included Jenny Altschuler, Sara Barratt, John Byng-Hall, Barbara Dale, Emilia Dowling, Sebastian Kraemer, Rob Senior, Renos Papadopoulos, and the late David Campbell, whom we all deeply miss. During the time we developed the courses, a number of other practitioners elsewhere in the United Kingdom also became interested in the links between family therapy and primary care, and joined up nationally to develop similar ideas. These included Hilary Graham, Dave Tomson, Jack Czauderna, Venetia Young, Sue Dickie – and Robert Mayer, whose loss we also mourn.

During that formative time, none of my own clinical and teaching work would have been possible without the exceptional multidisciplinary team at the Forest Road practice in Edmonton, north London, most importantly my long-standing GP partners Ron Singer, Mary Logan and Sally Jowett. They kept me going, along with the hundreds of people who saw me as patients. Necessarily anonymous here, they are the principal inspirations for the narrative in these pages. My work was also enhanced greatly by the psychologists who carried out collaborative work with me at Forest Road, either clinically or through research. These included Emilia Dowling and Alan Nance.

In more recent years, the team of teachers who have taught "Conversations Inviting Change" at the London Deanery (now part of Health Education England) have all made huge contributions to developing the approach, and in extending it to secondary health care and social care, as well as to team facilitation and conflict resolution. Active encouragement and resolute support for this came from Jonathan Burton, Neil Jackson and Tim Swanwick. Among the trainers who have been responsible for the work, I especially want to thank Helen Halpern, Lisa Miller, Serena North, Sarah Divall, Sue Elliott and Diana Kelly – as well as Nerys Cater, Christine Strickett and Sam Ferman for their administrative support (and with apologies to the many teachers and other staff there is insufficient space to mention here). The recent establishment of the Association of Narrative Practice in Healthcare (www.anph.org) has also created a highly creative forum for all of us, and provided further impetus for developments that are reflected in these pages.

As narrative-based practice has grown worldwide, it has been a special privilege to build up links with those pursuing similar work abroad, and to know some of the eminent thinkers in the field, including Rita Charon in the United States and Arthur Frank in Canada. I have greatly appreciated working alongside Maria Giulia Marini and Paola Chesi in Milan, Anat Gaver and Amnon Toledano in Israel, Pekka Larivaara in Finland, as well as Esperanza Diaz, Eivind Meland, Edvin Schei and their colleagues in Norway, Bent Stolberg and Bent Gyldenhof in Denmark, Akira Nakagawa and Akira Naito in Japan, and many other gifted and inspiring teachers elsewhere.

I have benefitted from the generosity of several friends and colleagues who have been willing to look at earlier drafts of this book – although its failings are self-evidently mine alone. For their thoughtful comments on different parts of the book (or in some cases, all of it), I want to thank Pooja Bhambra, Dariusz Galasiński, David Goosey, Jeremy Greenwood, Helen Halpern, Alasdair Honeyman, Lisa Miller and Julie Rooke.

As well as being a tactful and challenging reader, my wife Lee Wax has been unwavering in her love and in her encouragement to do the work that lies behind this book, and the book itself. It is dedicated to her and to our twins, who were born not long after "Conversations Inviting Change" first began, and are now about to go to university.

Foreword

John Launer is a friend, a fellow general practitioner and what might be termed a co-mentor. Our paths have crossed many times – as doctors, as scholars, as parents, as Londoners and more.

John is a fine storyteller himself, but his particular gift is helping others to tell and interpret their stories. Once or twice, when I have struggled with life's challenges, he has drawn a narrative of hope and healing out of me. Many times, we have (as doctors do, in professional confidence) exchanged anonymised stories about patients. What did these symptoms mean? How should I have reacted to this story fragment? What else should I have asked or offered? How should I respond next time the patient brings an update to his or her story? Always, John responded with more questions. Always, he enriched the narrative and inspired my clinical and moral imagination. He never told me what to do, and he never pretended that complex problems have simple or single answers. But through the wisdom of narrative conversations, I discovered options for taking seemingly unsolvable problems forward.

When I was very sick (in the middle of chemotherapy for cancer), John came to my house laden with treats and helped me construct what I later described as "the strangest story I have ever told" (Greenhalgh, 2017). While my medical prognosis was good (I had a small, treatable cancer that had not spread), in the early stages of my illness I was confused, frightened and suffused with (largely self-imposed) stigma. I discovered the truth in Arthur Frank's words: "A self that has become what it never expected to be requires repair, and telling autobiographical stories is a privileged means of repair" (Frank, 2000, p. 135).

As Bakhtin observed, it is impossible to craft a story without a listener. And to draw out the most productive stories, the listener must be open, interested, curious and imaginative. As John writes in his introductory chapter, the basis of all professional [clinical] practice is "attentive listening, careful inquiry, and the attempt to offer opportunities for easier and more creative narration." Sitting patiently beside me as I lay on the sofa, and saying remarkably little, John helped me make sense of what was happening and rebuild the strong, hopeful person it was happening to.

John has spent much of his professional lifetime developing a unique approach to training clinicians and therapists in the important but all-too-rare quality of active therapeutic listening. In this book, he describes his approach with numerous illustrative vignettes. These techniques are based on time-honoured and perhaps old-fashioned professional principles – but they are as important now as they have been down the centuries. I hope this book will be read widely and contribute to a renaissance of the narrative approach to clinical method.

Professor Trish Greenhalgh, Professor of Primary
Care Health Sciences, University of Oxford

References

Greenhalgh, T. (2017) Adjuvant chemotherapy: an autoethnography. *Subjectivity*. doi: 10.1057/s41286-017-0033-y

Frank, A.W. (2000) Illness and autobiographical work: dialogue as narrative destabilization. *Qualitative Sociology*, 23(1), 135–156.

Preface

This is a book about health and social care, and about stories. It describes an approach to everyday professional practice called "Conversations Inviting Change." The approach is based on a simple idea. *Everyone in health and social care – whether as a patient, service user, or practitioner – tells stories about their experiences, and can benefit from being skilfully questioned about them.*

The ideas in the book originate from a course at the Tavistock Clinic in London that Caroline Lindsey and I led for many years. Caroline had a background as a child psychiatrist, and I as a GP. We were both also trained as family therapists; in fact, Caroline had been my tutor. We strongly believed that narrative ideas and skills from the world of family therapy, if suitably adapted, could be useful in almost any professional encounter in primary health care (Launer, 1996a, 1996b). We thought the same skills could also be applied to peer supervision, training, management and team building. The original participants on our course included GPs, practice nurses, health visitors and community nurses, pharmacists and optometrists, and dentists (Launer and Lindsey, 1997). Caroline gave our approach the name "Conversations Inviting Change." The courses gave rise to a book called *Narrative-Based Primary Care: A Practical Guide* (Launer, 2002), the precursor of this one. Its aim was to make the ideas better known, so that people could try them out for themselves and integrate them into their existing forms of practice if they wished.

Once our course was well established, we started to receive requests to run workshops for groups of people elsewhere wanting to apply "Conversations Inviting Change" in their teaching and clinical practice and in supervision (Burton and Launer, 2003). Caroline retired, but a number of colleagues from different professional backgrounds who had completed our courses at the Tavistock became outstanding teachers of the approach. Together, we began to run trainings for the "London Deanery," the organisation that was responsible for postgraduate training of doctors in London at the time, and for developing their teachers and supervisors. We gradually transferred all our work there, and built up a multilevel system of training, ranging from one-day introductory workshops to extended courses where we taught more people to teach "Conversations Inviting Change" in their turn (London Deanery, 2012).

As we gained in experience, *we found that people who acquired narrative skills through doing peer supervision on our courses became more proficient in applying these to their work with patients and clients*. This became a central principle of our work. Hence, we focused on applying "Conversations Inviting Change" to workplace supervision (Launer, 2013). We also learned how to adapt everything we taught to contexts where people might have problems that everything we taught could be applied in any health care context – even ones that were highly complex technically, or more critical in terms of risk. We had to "get real" about the limits of narrative ideas and skills in situations where professionals or clients might have far more urgent needs than telling their stories, and where learners or colleagues might experience difficulties that required supervisors to do far more than listen and ask questions. We extended the use of the approach from training in peer supervision to applying it to team facilitation, conflict resolution, and to trainings in reflective practice and professionalism.

People from a far wider variety of professions became drawn to our courses. We extended our intake to include medical specialties right across the board, from transplant surgery to psychiatry, as well as nurses, allied health professionals, counsellors, managers, social workers and social work educators. The London Deanery itself became part of a national training organisation, Health Education England. As a result of all these developments, "Conversations Inviting Change" evolved from a fairly esoteric approach for a self-selected group of people to a mainstream supervision method taught across many professions. Invitations to run workshops and give presentations started to come in from all around the United Kingdom, and abroad. We demonstrated our approach and ran training workshops in Israel and Norway – and then in the United States, Canada, Japan and Australia, as well as widely around Europe. We found that the approach appeared to have cross-cultural value, possibly because stories are so universal, and a narrative-based approach made sense everywhere. In many of the places we have taught, the distinction between primary and secondary health care is not as sharp as it has been in the United Kingdom, and nor indeed is the division between health and social care.

We have now taught "Conversations Inviting Change" to several thousand practitioners in the United Kingdom and around the world. Almost everyone we teach recognises straight away how the skills can be applied in their own profession, discipline or specialty, and in their own work setting. The dilemmas we help people to address are not the province of any single profession. They are universal, across the professions. These dilemmas include:

- How do you practise when the authority of professionals, including doctors and social workers, can no longer be taken for granted?
- How can you share power with patients and clients, without letting go of evidence and best practice?

- How do you work alongside colleagues with other professions, views, beliefs and priorities?
- How can you practise humanely while following a huge agenda of risk assessment, targets and statutory duties?
- How can you hold on to optimism about the possibility of change, while seeing many people who are intractably distressed about their problems?
- How can you manage all of this when time and resources are so short, and organisational change is constant?
- How can you be a care professional and remain a caring person?

This book aims to address these questions. In an age when health and social care are becoming increasingly integrated, we believe there is an increasing need for "Conversations Inviting Change" across all the health and social care professions.

Notes on terminology

1 The terms "patient," "client" and "service user" all appear in this book, recognising that professionals in health and social care follow different kinds of usage, and that this is constantly changing. Wherever it is possible without causing confusion, we prefer the word "people" anyway. Likewise, the terms "practitioners" and "professionals" are both used to cover anyone working in health and social care, but the word "interviewer" also appears when referring to someone's role in holding effective conversations.
2 Some writers make a distinction between the words "story" and "narrative." We find it makes more sense to use them interchangeably. In practice, the main advantage of the word "narrative" is that it can be inflected into a verb ("to narrate," "narrating," etc.), conveying more of a sense of flow and dialogue. In some ways, our approach might be better described as "narrating-based."
3 Some readers will recognise many of the ideas and skills presented in this book as "systemic" just as much as "narrative-based." The similarities and distinctions between these terms are discussed in the Introduction.

References

Burton, J. and Launer, J. (eds) (2003) *Supervision and Support in Primary Care*. Abingdon: Radcliffe Medical Press.

Launer, J. (1996a) A social constructionist approach to family medicine. *Family Systems Medicine*, 13, 379–389.

Launer, J. (1996b) "You're the doctor, Doctor!" Is social constructionism a helpful stance in general practice consultations? *Journal of Family Therapy*, 18, 255–267.

Launer, J. (2002) *Narrative-Based Primary Care: A Practical Guide*. Abingdon: Radcliffe Medical Press.

Launer, J. (2013) Narrative-based supervision. In L.S. Sommers and J. Launer (eds), *Clinical Uncertainty in Primary Care: The Challenge of Collaborative Engagement*. New York: Springer, pp. 147–161.

Launer, J. and Lindsey, C. (1997) Training for systemic general practice: a new approach from the Tavistock Clinic. *British Journal of General Practice*, 47, 453–456.

London Deanery (2012) *Supervision Skills for Clinical Teachers: A World Class Teaching Initiative*. Available at: www.faculty.londondeanery.ac.uk/supervision-skills-for-clinical-teachers [accessed 17 May 2017].

Introduction
Narrative, health and social care

Key ideas in this chapter

- We experience, communicate and indeed create ourselves as individuals and human networks through the use of narratives or stories.
- Narrative ideas can provide a framework for thinking about everything that goes on in health and social care, including encounters with clients and between professionals.
- Health and social care professionals can make good use of such ideas and still remain grounded in the world of action and physical facts.
- Ideas from family therapy can act as a helpful bridge between narrative thinking from the social sciences, and the practical world of health and social care.
- Practitioners applying narrative-based approaches in health and social care can learn a great deal from each other in addressing the challenges involved.

Why narrative?

Storytelling is a defining human activity. Stories unite all cultures, cross all history, and arise in all circumstances. Stories in this sense are not fables, lies or fairy tales. They are the way we understand, experience, communicate and create meaning for ourselves, both as individuals and communities. They are the way we try to influence others, or assert our own positions in relation to theirs. The stories affect how people are seen, and how others tell stories about them in their turn. Stories are also dynamic: they constantly change as people tell them, and hear responses to them.

People generally come into contact with health and social care professionals because they have problems, but nearly always they present these problems by narrating them in a flow of words: "This happened, and then that happened, and I felt affected by it . . . I talked to some other people about it . . . Now I want to know what you think about it." In one sense, an account such as this is merely the way that people communicate their problems. In another sense, it is the story itself that needs attention. Whenever possible, they want to go away with a story that has a more helpful meaning for them: "I understand it better now . . . It all makes a bit more sense . . . I think I know what to do . . . I feel a bit different . . . "

Professionals tell stories to their clients too: "This is how I see your problem . . . This is what I think you should do about it . . . I hope that what I suggest will make things better . . . " Professional stories such as these are often connected to "official" narratives such as scientific evidence and public policy. Whatever the task, it is always embedded in a story for the client, and a story for the professional.

There are multiple opportunities in health and social care for service users to create new stories by sharing them with others. The same person may tell different stories to a receptionist, a practitioner and a passing cleaner – and will receive other proffered stories in exchange. None of these stories is definitive, nor are any of them distortions. Each is recreated in a different way, the outcome of the listener's role, identity, experience and power as much as the teller's.

Work settings offer similar opportunities for professionals to recreate narratives with each other too, as they exchange these in corridor conversations or team meetings. Thus, for clients and professionals alike, health and social care can be seen as spaces for the continual search for new and better meaning. Each time a story is told, or heard, or questioned, it changes. If the quality of the listening and the sensitivity of the questioning are well attuned, the change will be for the good.

A narrative-based approach sees attentive listening, careful inquiry, and the attempt to offer opportunities for easier and more creative narration as the basis of all professional work. Narrative ideas offer a conceptual framework for understanding all the different discourses – professional, scientific and political ones, together with lay or folk accounts of the world – that have to be integrated into everyday work. They can help practitioners to make sense of all the storytelling activities that they participate in with clients, colleagues, within teams, and throughout the health and social care services. Narrative ideas can also provide professionals with the skills to help themselves, along with clients and colleagues, to question, re-evaluate and continually adjust their own understanding.

Where the ideas come from

In the last part of the twentieth century, a wide range of academic and practical disciplines undertook what has generally been called a "narrative turn."

Broadly, one could describe this as a move from asking the question "what is *really* going on here?" to asking "how are people *giving an account* of their experiences?" This has happened in all kinds of fields: in psychology (Bruner, 1986; Roberts and Holmes, 1999), in the humanities (Ricoeur, 1984), and in the social sciences (Geertz, 1973). In all these subjects, the focus moved away significantly from observing the content of people's lives to examining the processes of living. These processes are characterised by speaking and thinking in a flow of words.

The world of narrative studies or narratology is now vast (Porter Abbott, 2008; Bal, 2009). People have studied how we construct our memories and our life stories in a similar way to authors writing novels: with time frames, characters and themes, and with elements such as plots and suspense. They have looked at how our stories change as time passes, and how they change as we have conversations with others. They have examined how we present ourselves to others in narrative form. They have described how stories change according to the power relationships between the people concerned, and the positions in which they wish to place themselves and their conversational partners (Harre and Moghaddam, 2003).

Many ideas about narrative have a "postmodern" flavour. Postmodernism rejects overarching accounts of reality (Lyotard, 1984). It challenges the idea that bodies of knowledge such as science, medicine or the law are purely objective. Instead, it understands all knowledge as the product of culture and of power: in other words, as stories that are accepted in any one time and place, but might one day cease to have meaning. Postmodernist thinkers reject the idea that exploring reality is like peeling away the layers of an onion, looking for the inner meaning concealed at the centre. Instead, they see it more like a tapestry of language that is continually being woven. This way of looking at language and reality is also related to the view described as *social constructionism* (Berger and Luckmann, 1966; Harre, 1986; McNamee and Gergen, 1992). Social constructionists believe that it is language that largely determines how we see reality, rather than the other way around.

Until relatively recently, there was very little interest in these ideas in the worlds of health and social care. Phrases such as "narrative studies," "postmodernism" or "social constructionism" meant nothing to most practitioners, unless they happened to work in academic departments. That has now changed, and it has changed radically. Partly this has come about because of social and political changes that have knocked the professions off their pedestals. Partly it is because of movements such as feminism and anti-racism that have invited people to look at their own beliefs and behaviour, and how these reflect their own vested interests. Consumerism has also had an effect. So have client pressure groups and disability rights activists. All these interest groups have different kinds of stories to offer, and they want to be heard. As a result, most health and social care professionals are now aware that few service users these days believe that what practitioners say or do is entirely objective or politically neutral. Professionals are coming to accept that they do not have a monopoly on describing people's experiences, or on telling them what to do about it. Our realities, in other words, have become contestable and open to negotiation.

Family therapy: a bridge between narrative, health and social care

Although narrative ideas have now taken hold in health and social care, there is another related field where they have been around for far longer – the field of family therapy, where the ideas set out in this book originated. To understand these more fully, it helps to know a little about the origins of family therapy, how it evolved, and how narrative ideas entered the field, before they spread to health and social care.

In its origins, family therapy drew largely on systems theory. This examines how parts of any system, human or otherwise, interact to affect each other. Family therapists were influenced by thinkers such as Gregory Bateson, a biologist whose theories explored the idea that everything in the living world is ultimately connected with everything else, through mutual influence or so-called "feedback loops" (Bateson, 1972). This means, for example, that you cannot really think about any single individual without considering the family members with whom they engage, as well as other important systems around them, including their community or workplace. The focus of family therapy is therefore on how people interact with each other, rather than how any particular individual feels and behaves. Because they look at the world in this way, family therapists often describe themselves as "systemic" therapists, or systemic practitioners. They generally work by seeing two or more people together – a couple or a family – and helping them to reflect on how they talk or deal with each other and with those around them. Equally, systemic practitioners usually take a lively interest in how different professionals or agencies interact, and how this impacts on the care of people and their families.

Over time, family therapists had to adapt their approach and their techniques to a world where they could no longer take notions such as objectivity and authority for granted. From fairly early on, they took social constructionist ideas on board. They largely moved away from theories that tried to explain what people and families *should* be like and how they *should* behave. Instead, they took the view that they needed to help people explore which ways of understanding the world made most sense for themselves, and how best to negotiate these with others. Increasingly, they have had to acknowledge the major effects of racial and other kinds of discrimination in their clients' lives, including gender issues (McGoldrick and Hardy, 2008; Burnham, 2011). They have had to take the religious beliefs of their clients into account. Family therapists have also turned their attention to their own beliefs and the power systems in which they operate. Probably more than other professions, they have tried to become aware of how their own practices and institutions can be oppressive, even with the best intentions. At the same time, they have tried to respect people's expectations that they should still have some expertise to offer, and that they should remain professional, ethical, competent, serious, and comply with the law.

In the last 20 years, family therapists have been particularly influenced by narrative ideas. This development is commonly associated with the Australian social worker and therapist Michael White. He emphasised the importance of the stories that people tell about themselves, and how these can evolve, or be "re-storied," as a result of therapeutic interventions (White and Epston, 1990; White, 2007). White's approach is known explicitly as "narrative therapy" and has been highly influential. Even practitioners who do not describe themselves as narrative therapists often base their work nowadays on the technique of asking creative questions, in order to invite people to construct new narratives (Dallos and Draper, 2010; McNab and Partridge, 2014). As a result, family therapists can often give other professionals in health and social care helpful guidance about how to apply narrative ideas and skills in their own work, especially in relation to holding therapeutic conversations.

"Systemic" and "narrative": what's the difference?

Since many people who train as family therapists come from health and social care, and often continue to work there, many words and ideas from family therapy have now entered those settings too. However, it is worth noting that the words "systemic" and "narrative" have acquired slightly different meanings in the world of health to that of social care. To avoid confusion, it is important to know about these differences.

Systemic ideas have affected social care a great deal. Many social workers are likely to have some understanding of what a "systemic" approach means, and how it differs from other, more individualised approaches, including psychoanalytic or behavioural ones. In their basic training, and subsequently, they may have heard about the way that systemic practitioners go about their work – for example, by interviewing a couple or a family together – and how this might be applied in social work, or when managing interagency work in social care (Fish et al., 2008; Goodman and Trowler, 2011; Munro, 2011). Conferences, courses and other activities related to systemic social work are now commonplace (Milowiz and Judy, 2013). In addition, some social care professionals, particularly in Australia and Canada, may be familiar with the specific practice of narrative therapy as introduced by Michael White, as described above. If the word "narrative" has resonances for them, it is likely to be specifically in connection with White's work and that of his followers, and its application in their own setting.

Within health care, perceptions of these terms are different. Doctors and health professionals may have some knowledge of systems theory, but this is far more likely to be in connection with physiological or organisational systems than with families. Most will be relatively unfamiliar with family therapy or the way the term "systemic" is used there. For doctors and nurses, the word also has an extraneous, and (in this context) rather unfortunate meaning: that of "intravenous"! Hence, they may find the term "systemic" puzzling in the context of human interactions. By contrast, they will generally feel much more comfortable with the word "narrative." They will connect this term not with Michael White or narrative therapy (which they are unlikely to have heard of), but with the emergence of a new movement known as "narrative medicine" (Greenhalgh and Hurwitz, 1998; Frank, 2001; Charon, 2006; Mehl-Madrona, 2007; Engel et al., 2008; Charon et al., 2016; Marini, 2016). This is a field that first developed around the turn of this century, coinciding with the early years of our own teaching of "Conversations Inviting Change."

Although narrative medicine drew on some of the same prior sources in the social sciences and elsewhere that inspired family therapists, it developed quite independently from the world of therapy. The mission of narrative medicine has been to restore humanity, imagination, and moral engagement to the medical world. It has asserted the importance of lived experience, and the recounting of that experience, in the face of the dominant intellectual voice in modern professional practice. This dominant voice often creates the impression that practice should be regulated only according to abstract principles or quantitative measurements. Narrative medicine encourages a commitment to what has been described as "narrative competence," including a literary-level sensitivity to the detailed content and contexts of every client's story (Montello, 1997; Charon, 2001; Grant, 2016). It acknowledges and respects scientific facts, but also emphasises how facts are narrated and acquire meaning in the minds of both practitioners and patients. It judges medical practice not just by successful technical outcomes, but also by whether it pays attention to the patient's story and contributes to one that is more cohesive and richer in meaning. A related concept is that of "narrative humility" (DasGupta, 2008), namely the capacity to acknowledge that people's stories are not objects to master, but dynamic accounts to engage with, while remaining open to their ambiguity, and engaging in constant self-evaluation about our own roles, expectations and responsibilities, and how the stories are affecting us personally.

Narrative medicine has now generated a tremendous variety of activities, including the study of literary texts and personal narratives of illness, as well as encouraging reflective writing by medical students (Kalitzkus and Matthiessen,

2009; Jones and Tansey, 2015). A similar movement is now emerging in social work, taking narrative as its basis, but without focusing exclusively on ideas from narrative therapy (Parton and O'Byrne, 2000; Milner, 2001; Riessman and Quinney, 2005; Roscoe et al., 2011; Gibson, 2012; Baldwin, 2013; Payne, 2014; Burack-Weiss et al., 2017).

Both narrative medicine and narrative social work are also closely aligned with the field known as narrative ethics (Charon and Montello, 2002; McCarthy, 2003; Wilks, 2005). In contrast to the abstract principles of traditional ethics, narrative ethics emphasises the importance of storytelling and listening, and on the role of professionals in conducting conversations ethically. According to this view, every juncture in a professional conversation is an opportunity for offering choices, so that clients can mould their own encounters with less direction or control by the professional. This can happen, for example, by inviting the client explicitly to choose which path to take (e.g. "Which aspect of the problem would you like to explore at this point?"). Instead of posing as a "fixer," the expert becomes a conversational partner. Clients can direct professionals towards what matters, and articulate what they actually want from the encounter. They can do so far more effectively than if the professional tries to second-guess these things for most of the conversation. "Choice" is therefore not just about decisions. It is embedded in every moment of every interaction (Launer, 2014, 2017). Where choices are genuinely constrained by statutory requirements, an approach guided by narrative ethics would also prompt the practitioner to be transparent about this, and to point out how and why the client's choices might be limited.

In its early years, we described "Conversations Inviting Change" as a systemic approach, but we found this caused puzzlement among doctors and health care professionals – so we changed to calling it a narrative-based approach. We do so not because it is derived from narrative therapy (it is not), but because it draws on the kinds of narrative ideas and skills that are widely used by all family therapists. We also do so because we feel our values are aligned with the narrative medicine movement, with the emerging movement of narrative social work, and with narrative ethics. At the same time, our work remains firmly rooted in systemic ideas, even though we do not often use the word.

Comparisons with coaching, counselling, motivational interviewing and CBT

Many health and social care professionals have had exposure to a variety of models and trainings in interactional skills before encountering narrative ideas. These include psychodynamic counselling, motivational interviewing, coaching, cognitive behavioural therapy, person-centred care and a variety of alternative approaches (Ronen and Freeman, 2007; Jacobs, 2010; Miller and Rolnick, 2013; Stewart et al., 2013; Rogers and Maini, 2016). Almost everyone who comes on a course in "Conversations Inviting Change" is curious to know the difference between such models and narrative-based practice.

What sets narrative practice apart from other approaches is its insistence on precise attentiveness to language, and on the idea that, wherever possible, the goals of any conversation should not be predetermined. It emphasises the need for conversations to be minutely responsive to the other person's self-expression from moment to moment, offers precise skills for doing so, and a closely choreographed and disciplined training methodology for helping people to acquire these skills. Another distinguishing feature is that we regard the whole range of belief systems and conversational frameworks that professionals apply as themselves forms of narrative, each imbued with certain assumptions related to their historical origins and the power relations they represent. For that reason, we encourage people to maintain a certain detachment and scepticism towards all these frameworks – including narrative-based practice itself. What ultimately matters is not whether any conversational model is applied slickly and consistently. It is whether the language of the practitioner arises out of the encounter itself, and is influenced as little as possible by prior prejudices, formulaic ways of working, or the unreflective application of professional dominance. This stance has been described as being "dogmatically undogmatic."

Interestingly, once people have had some exposure to narrative ideas and skills on our courses, some report how similar these seem to what they have learned from alternative frameworks, while others say it seems to challenge some of the cherished truths they have learned elsewhere. Paradoxically, one person may say they feel there is nothing new to learn because "this is identical to CBT/psychodynamic counselling/coaching/motivational interviewing, etc.," another may say they cannot adjust to a narrative approach because it questions their certainties, while a third person reports that they feel liberated because some of their reservations about other approaches have been confirmed!

A possible explanation for these diverse responses is that all effective approaches to conversational skills do share some commonalities, including an emphasis on positive regard and open questioning. Some people who use these spontaneously have therefore discovered for themselves the same kind of responsiveness that we teach. Others, by contrast, have learned to place more emphasis on more specific techniques such as goal-setting, active guidance or psychological interpretations, all of which we distinctly downplay in "Conversations Inviting Change." People's individual responses to what we teach may therefore reflect their own choices of how they have applied other models, rather than the models themselves.

Ultimately, almost everyone who acquires narrative-based skills finds ways of integrating these with other skills and techniques they already practise. Some do so only partially, for example by remaining largely within their previous modes of interaction, but adopting some narrative strategies that they find fit particularly well with these. Others develop ways of combining "Conversations Inviting Change" with approaches they have learned previously, in a syncretic fashion. Many decide to adopt narrative-based practice as an overall stance within which other ways of working can be offered with a lighter touch, or with more negotiability, and with a greater readiness to cede control of the conversation and move back to the client's own preferred trajectory if that turns out to be more appropriate.

Health and social care: differences and connectedness

In most teaching and writing, health and social care are treated as separate sectors. This is largely an arbitrary distinction. As every reader will know, many of the problems brought to one sector carry over into the other. One aim of this book is therefore to enable readers to help people working in one sector learn *about* those in the other, and *from* each other's work. A related aim is to indicate how frameworks such as narrative practice, or "Conversations Inviting Change," can serve both sectors equally, and help to bring them closer together.

In the United Kingdom and elsewhere, there is increasing convergence between the two sectors in organisational structures, funding streams and public policy. A similar convergence is happening with primary and secondary health care, and between social work and the wider world of social care. The boundaries between different fields are becoming more open to question. For example, many traditional hospital services are being moved into the community. Many of the responsibilities that social workers carried in the past are now commissioned from independent agencies, including private ones. In both health and social care, new roles and job titles appear each year (for example, "physician assistant" or "personal officer"). These are only a few examples of how the landscape is changing. Such developments pose challenges to existing professional identities – especially when they are associated with organisational upheaval and cost-cutting, as is often the case. Yet the trend is likely to be irreversible. Established professionals need to find ways of working with colleagues across old boundaries, and with new colleagues who may have different assumptions and expectations. Narrative practice may have its own contribution to make, by helping people to hear the different stories that people bring to their work, and how these stories change over time.

The descriptions and case vignettes in this book sometimes relate to identifiable professions, but elsewhere they simply refer to "practitioners," "professionals" or "interviewers" (see note on terminology in the Preface). This is intentional. Many of the issues that people in health and social care face in their work are not technical ones that only someone with the same training can help them to address. Far more often, they involve uncertainty, complexity or ethical dilemmas that could benefit from "talking through" with any other professional who is curious, sympathetic and suitably trained for this task, regardless of formal role. In the courses we have run over the years in "Conversations Inviting Change," some of the most exciting exchanges we have seen involved the most seemingly improbable of combinations: an anaesthetist supervising a counsellor, or a mental health social worker helping a medical education manager to reflect on a work problem. Seeing encounters such as this, and taking part in them, has helped to inspire the wide focus of this book. The variety of case vignettes are not present so that readers can seek out the ones that seem most obviously related to their own fields. Instead, they are there to demonstrate interprofessional similarities, and to indicate how much cross-fertilisation of ideas might be possible.

Challenges to narrative-based practice

The attractions of narrative ideas for health and social care professionals are clear. They offer a respectable intellectual framework for working in the twenty-first century – one that is no longer rooted in eighteenth-century mind/body dualism, or in Western individualism. They provide a single consistent way of thinking about all the different levels of their activity, including encounters with patients and clients, assessment, care planning, supervision, training, management work and political negotiation. They encourage us to question some of the apparently solid certainties of science and evidence. They offer a new view of such things as assessment and diagnosis, and sensitise practitioners to popular beliefs about illness and social deprivation. In addition, a narrative approach can help professionals to become more aware of their social and political roles. It encourages them to examine the power relations in their encounters with clients and with team members. It helps them to notice how power can be expressed in the subtleties of language, as well as in more obvious ways such as rudeness or paternalism. It can enrich their work by drawing their attention to the variety of cultures and beliefs with which they come into contact. It raises their awareness of gender, ethnicity and social class, including their own. It alerts them to the experiences of people living in adverse circumstances such as refugees. It can also assist them in letting go of a constant sense of responsibility for other people's problems, and in acquiring a greater sense of the possibilities open to the people they see in the course of their work.

If attractions of this kind of approach are numerous, so are the challenges. People expect professionals to be experts who can offer conventional explanations for their problems and deal with them accordingly. A narrative approach should help those working in health and social care to let go of rigid certainty about facts, but it should not make them so uncertain about everything that they feel unable to do their jobs. Professionals are not only paid to listen and speak. They also have to do things: to assess capacity, write care plans, mediate, advise, assess risk, take statutory action, stick needles into people, dispense drugs and carry out operations. They have to face disagreement, hostility and aggression. A narrative approach cannot ignore power relationships or exclude action. Nor can it be a licence for avoiding all the other normal professional tasks, such as giving advice, educating people, offering reassurance, assessing risks, or breaking bad news. It needs to fit a world where practitioners are regularly crossing over between different activities – such as helping with a marital or parenting problem and then having to make a court recommendation.

There is another obvious challenge. Most professionals have to work under tremendous pressure of time and workload. They face demands from managers and politicians, as well as resource shortages and constant organisational change. There is no point in trying to import narrative ideas and skills into everyday encounters if these only work in conversations lasting an hour, or when seeing people at regular intervals of every week or two, or by regularly inviting whole families to attend. Nor will they be helpful if they open up a "Pandora's box" that the interviewers do not have the skills or the resources to cope with.

One common first response of professionals when they encounter narrative-based practice for the first time is often: "In an ideal world we would use it, but it isn't possible given the kind of pressure we work under nowadays." They cite such constraints as limited consultation times, performance targets, standardised guidelines, the presence of computers and electronic record-keeping, along with wider problems of changing demographics among clients (including many who do not speak English and may need interpreters), as well as changing workforce patterns, including locum working. In addition, when people try out some of the techniques of narrative practice, they may find at first that it prolongs encounters. Very often, however, they later report that acquisition of a narrative-based stance leads to working that is not only faster, but actively assists most of the other tasks that need to be addressed in pressurised workplaces. It seems that a focus on the client's narrative from the outset creates trust and rapport, which then makes it possible for interviewers to address some of their official tasks such as record-keeping more transparently and efficiently. In the same way, approaching encounters with the conscious intention of paying attention to context (for example, cultural differences, the effects of translation or the transience of the professional relationship) makes it easier to take them into account and adjust to them than if these are regarded as obstacles to good practice. In the course of this book, there will be many examples to demonstrate how narrative-based practice can actually facilitate more effective working under pressure rather than adding extra unrealistic demands.

The "narrative turn" itself has also had its critics. Some have pointed out – with justice – that the term "narrative" is now used by different writers to describe everything from short spoken utterances to so-called "grand narratives" such as Marxism or neo-liberalism (Woods, 2011). Others have drawn attention to the tendency of narrative scholars to place an emphasis on Western middle-class constructions in place of culturally diverse ones (Saville-Troike, 1989), on long-term instead of episodic experience (Strawson, 2004), on good stories in preference to deceitful or manipulative ones (Gabriel, 2004), and on language at the expense of other forms of expression, including body language and silence (Sartwell, 2000). In spite of this, narrative theorists have, by and large, been able to hold on to their positions through accommodating to these critiques, and by promoting the strengths of their defining stance, rather than trying to defend specific articles of faith.

The biggest challenge in taking a narrative approach is knowing when to stop. Disease, disability, deprivation and death are not "just stories." Although they may be open to different interpretation by different individuals and cultures, they each rest on a bedrock of incontestable reality. Professionals who get carried away by narrative ideas to the point where they forget this are not safe (Launer, 1996). Knowledge applied uncritically can lead to abuses of power, but pursuing narratives without a sense of realism can be literally fatal. Narrative ideas can help people question their own convictions, but no one should play linguistic games with people's lives.

The approach described in this book is an attempt to address all these challenges. It tries to do justice to a complex and sophisticated body of contemporary thought, while also paying respect to the realities of life in the health and social services. It imports some quite difficult concepts and techniques, without overloading busy professionals with excessively abstract theories or with jargon. The overriding intention is to present ideas in a way that is accessible and applicable. The aim is to bring them into routine work in a way that enables practitioners and shares more power with clients. When the book refers to therapy, this does not imply formal sessions, nor working with whole families. It means therapy in its literal sense: a form of healing.

This is emphatically a book about *practice*, specifically about the use of "Conversations Inviting Change." It does not give a detailed account of narrative theory, of the kind you might find in textbooks of social science, nor does it explain how to use literary texts to enhance professional training or sensitivity. It contains no guidance about carrying out narrative research into the stories that patients and/or professionals tell and write. Instead, this book is about how practitioners and their clients can create richer meaning in their encounters. It chiefly addresses the question "How do we speak (or not speak), and what do we do (or not do) from moment to moment, if we understand the world as constructed to a significant degree by the stories that we and other people tell each other?"

References

Bal, M. (2009) *Narratology: Introduction to the Theory of Narrative*, 3rd edn. Toronto: University of Toronto Press.

Baldwin, P. (2013) *Narrative Social Work: Theory and Application*. Bristol: Policy Press.

Bateson, G. (1972) *Steps to an Ecology of Mind*. New York: Ballantine.

Berger, P. and Luckmann, T. (1966) *The Social Construction of Reality*. London: Allen Lane.

Bruner, J. (1986) *Actual Minds, Possible Worlds*. Cambridge, MA: Harvard University Press.

Burack-Weiss, A., Lawrence, S.L. and Mijangos, L.B. (2017) *Narrative in Social Work Practice: The Power and Possibility of Story*. New York: Columbia University Press.

Burnham, J. (2011) Developments in social GRRRAAACCEEESSS: visible – invisible and voiced – unvoiced. In I.-B. Krause (ed.), *Culture and Reflexivity in Systemic Psychotherapy: Mutual Perspectives*. London: Karnac, pp. 139–160.

Charon, R. (2001) Narrative medicine: a model for empathy, reflection, profession and trust. *Journal of the American Medical Association*, 286(15), 1897–1902.

Charon, R. (2006) *Narrative Medicine: Honoring the Stories of Illness*. Oxford: Oxford University Press.

Charon, R. and Montello, M. (eds) (2002) *Stories Matter: The Role of Narrative in Medical Ethics*. New York: Routledge.

Charon, R., DasGupta, S., Hermann, N., Irvine, C., Marcus, E.R., Riviera Colòn, E., et al. (2016) *The Principles and Practice of Narrative Medicine*. Oxford: Oxford University Press.

Dallos, R. and Draper, R. (2010) *An Introduction to Family Therapy: Systemic Theory and Practice*, 3rd edn. Maidenhead: McGraw-Hill.

DasGupta, S. (2008) Narrative humility. *Lancet*, 371, 980–981.

Engel, J.D., Zarconi, J., Pethel, L.L. and Missimi, S.A. (2008) *Narrative in Health Care: Healing Patients, Practitioners, Profession and Community*. Abingdon: Radcliffe.

Fish, S., Munro, E. and Bairstow, S. (2008) *SCIE Report 19: Learning Together to Safeguard Children. Developing a Multi-Agency Systems Approach for Case Reviews*. Available at: www.scie.org.uk/publications/reports/report19.asp [accessed 17 May 2017].

Frank, A. (2001) Experiencing illness through storytelling. In S. Tooms (ed.), *Handbook of Phenomenology and Medicine*. New York: Springer, pp. 229–245.

Gabriel, Y. (2004) The voice of experience and the voice of the expert – can they speak to each other? In B. Hurwitz, T. Greenhalgh and V. Skultans (eds), *Narrative Research in Health and Illness*. London: Blackwell, pp. 168–185.

Geertz, C. (1973) *The Interpretation of Cultures*. New York: Basic Books.

Gibson, M. (2012) Narrative practice and social work education: using a narrative approach in social work practice education to develop struggling social work students. *Practice*, 24(1), 53–65.

Goodman, S. and Trowler, I. (2011) *Social Work Reclaimed: Innovative Frameworks for Child and Family Social Work*. London: Jessica Kingsley.

Grant, A. (2016) Narrative competence: a neglected area in undergraduate curricula. *Nursing Education Today*, 36, 7–9.

Greenhalgh, T. and Hurwitz, B. (1998) *Narrative Based Medicine: Dialogue and Discourse in Clinical Practice*. London: BMJ Books.

Harre, R. (ed.) (1986) *The Social Construction of Emotions*. Oxford: Blackwell.

Harre, R. and Moghaddam, F.M. (eds) (2003) *The Self and Others: Positioning Individuals and Groups in Personal, Political and Cultural Contexts*. Westport, CT: Greenwood.

Jacobs, M. (2010) *Psychodynamic Counselling in Action*, 4th edn. London: Sage.

Jones, E.M. and Tansey, E.M. (eds) (2015) *The Development of Narrative Practices in Medicine c.1960–c.2000: Welcome Witnesses to Contemporary Medicine*, vol. 52. London: Queen Mary University of London.

Kalitzkus, V. and Matthiessen, P. (2009) Narrative-based medicine: potential, practice and pitfalls. *The Permanente Journal*, 13(1), 80–86.

Launer, J. (1996) "You're the doctor, Doctor!" Is social constructionism a helpful stance in general practice consultations? *Journal of Family Therapy*, 18, 255–267.

Launer, J. (2014) Patient choice and narrative ethics. *Postgraduate Medical Journal*, 90, 484.

Launer, J. (2017) Narrative ethics in primary care. In A. Papanikitas and J. Spicer (eds), *Handbook of Primary Care Ethics*. Milton Keynes: CRC, pp. 259–265.

Lyotard, J.-F. (1984) *The Post Modern Condition: A Report on Knowledge*. Minneapolis, MN: University of Minnesota Press.

Marini, M.G. (2016) *Narrative Medicine: Bridging the Gap Between Evidence-Based Care and the Medical Humanities*. New York: Springer.

McCarthy, J. (2003) Principlism or narrative ethics: must we choose between them? *Journal of Medical Ethics: Medical Humanities*, 29, 65–71.

McGoldrick, M. and Hardy, V. (2008) *Re-Visioning Family Therapy: Race, Culture and Gender in Clinical Practice*, 2nd edn. New York: Guilford Press.

McNab, S. and Partridge, K. (eds) (2014) *Creative Positions in Adult Mental Health: Outside-In, Inside-Out*. London: Karnac.

McNamee, S. and Gergen, K. (eds) (1992) *Therapy as Social Construction*. London: Sage.

Mehl-Madrona, L. (2007) *Narrative Medicine: The Use of History and Story in the Healing Process*. Rochester, VT: Bear & Company.

Miller, W.R. and Rollnick, S. (2013) *Motivational Interviewing: Helping People Change*. New York: Guilford Press.

Milner, J. (2001) *Women and Social Work: Narrative Approaches*. Basingstoke: Palgrave Macmillan.

Milowiz, W. and Judy, M. (2013) *Systemic Social Work Throughout Europe*. Available at: www.asys.ac.at/step/zpapers/STEP%20manual%20mc2.pdf [accessed 17 May 2017].

Montello, M. (1997) Narrative competence. In H.L. Nelson (ed.), *Stories and Their Limits: Narrative Approaches to Bioethics*. London: Routledge, pp. 185–197.

Munro, E. (2011) *The Munro Review of Child Protection: Final Report. A Child-Centred System*. London: Department for Education. Available at: www.education.gov.uk/munroreview/downloads/8875_DfE_Munro_Report_TAGGED.pdf [accessed 17 May 2017].

Parton, N. and O'Byrne, P. (2000) *Constructive Social Work: Towards a New Practice*. Basingstoke: Macmillan.

Payne, M. (2014) Strengths, narrative and solution practice. In M. Payne, *Modern Social Work Theory*, 4th edn. Basingstoke: Palgrave Macmillan, pp. 243–270.

Porter Abbott, H. (2008) *The Cambridge Introduction to Narrative*, 2nd edn. Cambridge: Cambridge University Press.

Ricoeur, P. (1984) *Time and Narrative: Volume 1*. Chicago, IL: University of Chicago Press.

Riessman, C.K. and Quinney, L. (2005) Narrative in social work: a critical review. *Qualitative Social Work*, 4(4), 319–412.

Roberts, G. and Holmes, J. (eds) (1999) *Narrative in Psychiatry and Psychotherapy*. Oxford: Oxford University Press.

Rogers, J. and Maini, A. (2016) *Coaching For Health: Why It Works and How to Do It*. Maidenhead: Open University Press.

Ronen, T. and Freeman, A. (eds) (2007) *Cognitive-Behaviour Therapy in Clinical Social Work Practice*. New York: Springer.

Roscoe, K.D., Carson, A.M. and Madoc-Jones, L. (2011) Narrative social work: conversations between theory and practice. *Journal of Social Work Practice*, 25(1), 47–61.

Sartwell, C. (2000) *End of Story: Towards an Annihilation of Language and History*. Albany, NY: State University of New York Press.

Saville-Troike, M. (1989) *The Ethnography of Communication: An Introduction*, 2nd edn. Oxford: Blackwell.

Stewart, M., Brown, J.B., Weston, W. and McWhinney, I.R. (2013) *Patient-Centred Medicine: Transforming the Clinical Method*, 3rd edn. Abingdon: CRC Press.

Strawson, G. (2004) Against narrativity. *Ratio*, 17(4), 428–452.

White, M. (2007) *Maps of Narrative Practice*. New York: Norton.

White, M. and Epston, D. (1990) *Narrative Means to Therapeutic Ends*. New York: Norton.

Wilks, T. (2005) Social work and narrative ethics. *British Journal of Social Work*, 35(8), 1249–1264.

Woods, A. (2011) The limits of narrative: provocations for the medical humanities. *Medical Humanities*, 37(2), 73–78.

CHAPTER ONE

Narrative practitioners at work

> **Key ideas in this chapter**
>
> - There is a usually a tension present in professional encounters between the storytelling that the patient or client brings, and the practitioner's need for pattern recognition, action and closure.
> - Narrative practice aims to integrate these as harmoniously as circumstances allow.
> - This involves close attentiveness and responsiveness to language, and to the contexts that make sense of the words being used.
> - It also involves offering others choices about how to make use of the practitioner, and about how to proceed at each juncture in the conversation.
> - Professional power is a feature of every encounter, but self-aware practitioners can monitor this and manage it ethically.

Introduction

If you observe professionals interacting with their clients, you will nearly always observe some kind of struggle going on between two styles of conversation. This can be described as a tension between "narrative" and "normative" styles. (I have adapted this from Jerome Bruner's (1990) distinction between narrative and "logico-scientific" discourses.)

Clients who use health and social care, by and large, have a story to tell. If you want to find out how powerful the storytelling drive is, you have only to interrupt them prematurely in their narratives – and to notice how they generally carry on from exactly where they left off. Sometimes the stories will be very clear. At other times, these may be hesitant, disjointed, fragmented, complicated, punctuated by silence, or full of things that are puzzling. Nevertheless, the flow of words will almost certainly resemble some kind of story, with characters, events, trouble, and a timeline.

While clients want to express the uniqueness of their experiences, professionals generally try to do the opposite: to find the common denominators in these stories, and then to move towards an action or conclusion as rapidly as possible. Our utterances are therefore largely aimed at matching others' words against patterns of description, standards, or norms. They may be norms of entitlement ("Does this person fit the criteria for the service they are requesting?"), norms of risk ("Do I need to take action?"), or norms related to a wide range of legal, scientific or administrative categories. Although a few clients are in a hurry and only want their professionals to get on with the task (and conversely, professionals can be overcome by curiosity and forget about time constraints), the great majority of work encounters are characterised by an attempt by one party to tell a story, and an attempt by the other party to take an essentially norm-based or *normative* stance in order to identify what decisions or actions seem necessary.

Health and social care workers seem to vary greatly in their awareness of this tension. Some exert their professional power unthinkingly and as a matter of routine, ensuring that the normative style dominates every consultation. Effectively, they screen each person's words for whatever corresponds to their own conceptual framework ("falls," "hitting," "bad memory"), and conveniently tune out anything else, in order to move towards a decision or determination of some kind. The professional's normative approach may be so dominant that it takes over the encounter completely. By contrast, some professionals are more tolerant of narratives. They may pay attention, perhaps out of empathy, in the opening part of the meeting. Nevertheless, they may often have difficulty sustaining this throughout the encounter, and will bring the normative style into play as soon as they think it polite enough to do so, thus foreclosing opportunities for clients to develop their own stories further.

Taking a narrative-based stance

While it is possible to manage any professional encounter by taking a purely normative approach, it is also possible to follow a client's cues in a way that allows far fuller expression of their stories *and* leads to better decision-making. This is what it means to take a narrative-based stance. Box 1.1 gives a very brief illustration of the difference between a purely normative approach and a narrative-based one, using a fictional scenario: two different occupational therapists carrying out a home assessment for mobility aids, in the same patient.

Box 1.1 Normative and narrative-based approaches during a home assessment

Therapist A (taking a normative approach)

Therapist A: Well, as you know, I've come to look at your home because of your falls.

Client: I've had a lot of them lately.

Therapist A: Yes, your social worker mentioned that. So let's go round and look at what we can do for you.

Therapist B (using a narrative-based stance)

Therapist B: Well, as you know, I've come to look at your home because of your falls.

Client: Yes, I've had a lot of them lately.

Therapist B: Did anything cause this, do you think?

Client: Oh, I thought the social worker would have told you. My son used to live here and always helped me get around.

Therapist B: Is he not here any more?

Patient: No, that's the terrible thing. He got killed in a car accident . . .

Although the opening of the conversation in Box 1.1 is the same each time, the two occupational therapists go in entirely different directions. Therapist A remains incurious about anything except her own task, whereas Therapist B tries to understand the personal context that has made the task necessary. To do so, she actively *tracks* the language used by the client, picking up the signal that the son "used to live here" in order to deepen her inquiry. By the end of the conversation, each of the therapists may have reached the same point – in the technical sense of which mobility aids to recommend – or they may not. The more attentive one may decide to address other needs in addition. These might cover, for example, meeting her client's psychological needs, advising her where she might get support for these, or arranging more practical help in the home.

Box 1.2 shows the same contrast between the two approaches, this time based on genuine transcripts of two different medical consultations with real patients. It is taken from a famous paper by the US sociologist Eliot Mishler and his colleagues (Mishler et al., 1989). It illustrates how professionals can either unthinkingly set limits to the narrative, or choose to pay attention to it. In the first consultation, a doctor ignores signals of uncertainty and anxiety to such a gross extent that the patient is effectively reduced to tears. In the second consultation, another far more attentive doctor manages to listen to a patient's narrative in a more precise way, and to use it as a cue to inquire about something of medical importance – a witness account of a seizure the patient has suffered. It is worth examining these short extracts closely, to identify what is typical of a normative interview, and to contrast it with a more narrative approach.

Box 1.2   Normative and narrative-based approaches in two medical consultations

Doctor A ignores a patient's words

Patient: It's one spot right here. It's real sore. But then there's like pains in it. Ya-know how . . . I don't know what it is.

Doctor: Okay . . . Fevers or chills?

Patient: No.

Doctor: Okay. Have you been sick to your stomach, or anything like that?

Patient: [Sniffles, crying] I don't know what's going on.

Doctor B pays attention to a patient's words and uses them to seek important information (a witness account of a seizure)

Patient: My boss hadn't got all the parts for it, so I started working on another car, ya-know? That's when I ended up having the seizure.

Doctor: Okay . . . So did your boss or someone else see the seizure happen?

What is striking in the first example in Box 1.2 is that the doctor fails to hear the crucial words "I don't know what it is" or chooses to ignore them. Instead, he focuses only what he believes matters to him as a physician, namely to progress through a litany of possible symptoms. As a result, the patient's anxiety escalates further. Paradoxically, this upsets the patient so much that it makes the doctor's task of taking a history even harder. In the second example, by contrast, the doctor appears to pay attention to the words of the story and visualise the exact scene being described. This not only results in the patient being heard, but opens up an opportunity for the doctor to seek exactly what he needs from a technical point of view: a detailed, objective account of the seizure from an observer.

From these illustrations, the advantages of taking an approach led by the narrative should be clear. A narrative-based approach:

- is respectful to the client;
- allows others to talk more freely and follow their own logical flow;
- allows professionals to calibrate their speech to the client's world view, degree of understanding, and preferred kind of conversation;
- gives space for people to focus on the major events and themes of their lives;
- can facilitate disclosure of important information; and
- can lead to decision-making and advice that is better informed and matched to the client.

Given these obvious advantages, why is the normative style so dominant in professional conversations? There are in fact some more or less universal obstacles that stand in the way of professionals using a narrative approach as their preferred one. These are:

- An ingrained belief, inculcated during training and reinforced by professional culture, that all encounters with clients are solely about making decisions and taking action.
- Care that is led by management or financial models that appear to carry more authority or objectivity than human values.
- A conviction that decisions and actions can only be achieved through a normative approach, especially if time is limited.
- A lack of appropriate micro-skills to elicit significant factual information through a narrative approach.
- No previous training in how to reach decisions and actions collaboratively through working with the narrative.

One of the chief aims of "Conversations Inviting Change" is to overcome these obstacles and to equip professionals with the narrative micro-skills to let go of them and integrate normative information-gathering and decision-making within a narrative-based approach whenever possible.

Sustaining a narrative approach

Narrative-based practice works not just for the opening of an encounter. Nor does it mean seizing on elements of the narrative that offer opportunities for nudging clients in the desired direction (something we see very commonly on training courses, and that we describe as "narrative-based manipulation"). Instead, it means regarding *every* juncture in the conversation as a potential opportunity for offering a choice about how to move forward, so that clients genuinely create their own stories and are no longer controlled by the professional. This happens mainly by noticing a cue and testing its potential for narrative development.

Boxes 1.3 and 1.4 show extracts from two interviews, carried out by a social worker and a nurse, respectively, where each is applying narrative-based practice and sustaining this through the length of the conversation. Notice how the practitioners manage to follow the words of the patient or client closely and match their responses accordingly, while at the same time applying appropriate professional judgement and fulfilling their expected tasks.

Box 1.3   A social worker visits a mother whose son is on a child protection plan

Social worker:	I've heard from the school that Michael's attendance is much better, and I can see you've done a lot to make the home much safer.
Mother:	Thanks. I've got myself together a bit more, and he's a lot happier, I think.
Social worker:	You have, haven't you. Do you know what's helped you to do that?
Mother:	I think I just got determined to show everyone. I was so busy trying to get by, and I did feel a bit down.
Social worker:	So how are you feeling now in general?
Mother:	Better. I do still get a bit down, but I guess I'm not letting it really get to me like before.
Social worker:	Is it OK if I ask you a bit about the times when you still feel bit down?
Mother:	Yes, I guess it's loneliness a lot of the time.
Social worker:	How has the loneliness come about?
Mother:	Well, I moved down here originally because of a job offer, but then they made me redundant, so I ended up living somewhere I didn't really know anybody.
Social worker:	Is that still the case?
Mother:	Not so much now. I thought of going back up north to my family, but now my sister's moved down here too.
Social worker:	Will that make a difference, do you think?
Mother:	Yes, quite a lot. She and Michael are really close, and I can get a bit of a break sometimes.
Social worker:	That sounds good. How do you think things are going to go from here?

| Mother: | I know I'll have my ups and downs. But the child protection stuff was a real jolt for me, and I've talked to my sister a lot about it. I don't think things are ever going to go back to where they were. |
| Social worker: | I can hear you're pretty determined they won't. From all I can see, you do seem to be well on the way to achieving the targets for avoiding any proceedings, and I'm happy at this stage to give a much more positive report to the next case conference. |

Box 1.4   A nurse sees a patient with a sore throat

Patient: I've got a sore throat.

Nurse: Tell me about it.

Patient: I'm surprised how painful an ordinary sore throat can be.

Nurse: Is it quite unusual for you to have this kind of thing?

Patient: It's not just that. I'm concerned the pain has lasted so long.

Nurse: That's not uncommon, but if it's your first it can be a bit of a shock. Are there any particular concerns you have about it?

Patient: Well, maybe I'm being a complete hypochondriac, but I've heard that heart trouble can make your throat hurt.

Nurse: Your symptoms sound quite different, but are there other things making you worry it's your heart?

Patient: Apart from my throat, nothing else is hurting.

Nurse: Is there any other reason you might worry about heart disease?

Patient: Yes, my father had a lot of heart trouble and he died from a heart attack last year. He was only 49.

Nurse: I'm really sorry. What impact do you think that's had on you?

Patient: It's made me nervous that the same sort of thing is going to happen in my case.

Nurse: Are there things we can do to help you find out, or prevent it happening?

Patient: I'd never really thought of that. It certainly wasn't why I came today.

Nurse: No, but we might be able to deal with the sore throat now and bring you back to check out your risks of heart disease.

Patient: To be honest, I'm not entirely sure I want to go into that. If it's in my genes, I'd rather not know.

Nurse: So should I try and offer you some screening tests like a cholesterol check, or should I back off?

Patient: That's an interesting question. I guess your job is to persuade people to have their cholesterol measured.

Nurse: Not exactly. My job is to offer it. It's up to you to choose whether you want me to.

Patient: I guess it would make sense for me to come back and get these things sorted out.

Nurse: I'd certainly be happy to do that.

Patient: But in the meantime, what can you do about my sore throat?

Nurse: Mainly giving advice and reassurance. Gargling with salt water may help. And it'll probably go by itself in a few days.

Patient: So when should I book an appointment to get the other stuff sorted?

Nurse: How does two weeks sound?

Patient: Two weeks sounds fine.

As these conversations both show, one of the most challenging tasks in the whole of health and social care may be to manage each encounter so that it continually meets both narrative and normative requirements. This means recognising the equal legitimacy of the client's need for self-expression *and* one's own need to achieve pattern recognition, action, including adherence to guidelines and protocols, and closure. It means finding ways to satisfy both needs at every moment in the conversation. In other words, the professional has to try to bring normative questions or statements into the conversation at moments that fit in with the natural flow of the other person's story as well.

Figure 1.1 is a schematic diagram showing the integration of narrative and normative approaches, based on the traditional depiction of "yin" and "yang" in Chinese thought (Foell, 2017).

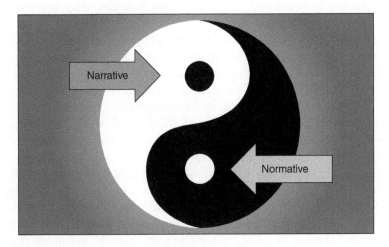

Figure 1.1   Integrating narrative and normative approaches

As well as the complementarity between the two approaches, note how each contains an element of the other. The standards or norms of health and social work that have to be embedded in professional conversations can themselves be regarded as types of official narrative, while conversely the narratives that people present to practitioners are also forms of evidence that can contribute towards the actions or decisions that emerge from these conversations.

Power and reflexivity

Sharing power is at the heart of a narrative approach. Every technique is aimed at helping the client to lead the narrative wherever possible, and to participate in the choices and dilemmas that have to be addressed. Sharing power is not just about sharing the final decision about what to do. It is about looking for opportunities at every moment in the consultation to hand over power. Nowhere is this more important than in the minute-to-minute conduct of the consultation itself. In some ways, it is still very countercultural for interviewers to ask patients to make decisions in this way. It requires an ability to observe one's own role in an interaction and to comment on this freely to the patient. This skill calls for a certain level of sophistication, and a degree of confidence.

At the same time, in virtually all encounters in health and social care, the professional does actually have more power than the client or patient. This is not only because professionals have expert knowledge, and the authority to permit or refuse access to a vast range of resources, including prescription medicines, hospital referral and state benefits. Professionals are also very often representatives of a dominant cultural group in terms of social class, ethnicity, sexuality, gender or in other ways. It is usually the professionals who, in the last resort, can say how things should be organised, what the limits of negotiation are, and how the encounter itself should be conducted.

While professionals who use a narrative-based approach should be looking for opportunities throughout every conversation to share power, they also need to be aware that few clients will feel that the encounter is a totally equal one. For this reason, enacting narrative-based practice involves more than following cues and asking good questions. Attentiveness and responsiveness to language are prerequisites for such practice but are not enough by themselves. As the case examples above show, it also requires ethical commitment, emotional engagement, and political and social awareness. It may also require (among other things) spontaneity, humour and risk-taking – including speaking bluntly rather than beating around the bush, or alternatively by accepting a client's anger as a legitimate form of expression rather than a threat. Practitioners also need to be alert to when the other party in the conversation appears to be constrained – either by their context in which it is taking place (for example, the statutory framework or institution), the unavoidable differentials of power in the relationship, or by the general anxiety that nearly always accompanies seeing a health or social care professional in the first place.

What we have found matters above all is an awareness of self – both personal and professional, as well as political in its broadest sense – and a willingness to reflect at any moment on what one is saying and why, and to observe its effects on the inter-action. This self-awareness, which also encompasses attentiveness to the contexts influencing the conversations, is sometimes termed "reflexivity." It implies "having a self-conscious account of the production of knowledge as it is being produced" (Baarts et al., 2000). In other words, a narrative stance involves not only paying attention to the other person, but also to oneself and the interaction as a whole, to see how well the parties are managing to generate forms of meaning and action that are acceptable to both of them. It means cultivating the ability to contribute to the new story while at the same time tracking its progress through one's own and the client's contributions, and the interaction between the two. It also means taking into account the complex and multilayered social contexts in which encounters take place, while still remaining engaged and safe (Iedema, 2011). Reflexivity also means taking responsibility for restraint in the use of professional power: for example, not imposing narratives that reflect the view of a particular gender, ethnic group or profession – but equally in stating transparently when action needs to be taken.

In many circumstances, reflexivity involves paying attention to silence as well as utterances. Every silence is a communication, open to readings and misreadings, to appropriate responses or inappropriate ones. Some clients prefer not to speak at length about their experiences, and practitioners need to adjust their own responses accordingly. Even interviewers who become skilled in using "Conversations Inviting Change" will inevitably find that there are some clients, students and col-leagues for whom the approach absolutely does not work. For whatever reason, it signifies something to them that they find off-putting or unnatural. In instances such as these, practitioners need to be able to adjust their own belief that their favoured approach to professional conversations will suit everyone. Every skill and technique described in this book can be applied with thoughtfulness and com-passion, or in a mechanical or dominating way. There is certainly no guarantee that it will turn an insensitive professional into a sensitive one, and in our teaching work we have sometimes had students who were convinced they had mastered the approach, when our own perception was that they had merely co-opted a few techniques into their own pre-existing paternalistic styles of consultation.

Many readers might recognise that they already apply reflexivity, although they might use different words to describe it. However, naming this as a profes-sional responsibility seems to help professionals to become both more involved and more detached in the process of co-creating stories. This is not the paradox it may seem. Practitioners become more involved in their work, in the sense of staying close to what their clients are telling them or asking them. At the same time, they also become more detached, through watching the effect of their own proffered questions or stories, and through their increased ability to change these in response to what they hear.

Suggested exercises

1 After an encounter with a client, compare the final story with the initial one that the patient brought. How was it different? How far was it a normative one and what other elements did it have?
2 Try to recall how you managed limitations of time or resources, or indicated them. To what extent did tracking the narrative lengthen the conversation, and to what extent did it help it to progress?
3 In any conversation with a client, pay attention to the first juncture when you asked a question. Afterwards, think about why you chose that juncture. What then happened? What other questions could you have asked? What might have happened if you had?
4 Try to pay attention to how long you maintain a narrative stance in an encounter with clients, when you change over to a more normative one, and why.

References

Baarts, C., Tulinius, C. and Reventlow, S. (2000) Reflexivity: a strategy for a patient-centred approach in general practice. *Family Practice*, 17, 430–434.

Bruner, J. (1990) *Acts of Meaning: Four Lectures on Mind and Culture*. Cambridge, MA: Harvard University Press.

Foell, J. (2017) *Personal communication*.

Iedema, R. (2011) Creating safety by strengthening clinicians' capacity for reflexivity. *Quality and Safety in Health Care*, 20(S1), i80–i86.

Mishler, E., Clark, J.A., Ingelfinger, J. and Simon, P. (1989) The language of attentive patient care: a comparison of two medical interviews. *Journal of General Internal Medicine*, 4, 325–335.

CHAPTER TWO

Concepts
The "seven C's"

Key ideas in this chapter

- Practitioners can benefit from a simple framework of concepts to guide then in taking a narrative-based approach.
- "Conversations Inviting Change" offers such an approach, using seven words beginning with the letter C.
- The fundamental reorientation for taking a narrative-based approach involves seeing the world in terms of dynamic and interactive processes rather than static or linear ones.
- It also involves seeing professional conversations as shared acts of creation between someone with a problem and someone else with expert knowledge and skills.

Introduction

Most professionals embarking on a narrative approach find it useful to learn a simple conceptual framework at the outset. Over time, we have developed one for "Conversations Inviting Change." It is based on seven words all beginning with C. Of course, one could just as well summarise a narrative approach with eight words beginning with S, or 11 with P, and so forth. What matters are not the specific words, but the attitude that they evoke. They serve as a simple summary of complex ideas, providing a mantra for learners who want to practise a narrative approach, rather than a toolkit or a "do-it-yourself" guide. The cases described in this chapter are from participants on our courses and workshops, and other narrative practitioners. Every story, here and elsewhere, has been heavily disguised (or several stories combined) to prevent anyone accidentally recognising the people involved.

The seven concepts we emphasise in "Conversations Inviting Change" are:

- conversations;
- curiosity;
- contexts;
- complexity;
- challenge;
- caution; and
- care.

The sections that follow explore each of the seven concepts in more detail. A summary appears in Box 2.1 at the end of the chapter.

Conversations

A narrative approach sees conversations in a particular way: not as a vehicle for an intervention, but as interventions in their own right. This means seeing the conversational process itself as therapeutic. It involves moving away from the idea of problem-solving and towards the idea of "problem dissolution." The main way this happens in the course of conversations is by inviting others to consider their problems from new perspectives. Such invitations may come in the suggestion that something can be given a name, diagnosis or formulation. It may involve an intervention such as direct advice about where to turn for help, or an onward referral. It may arise principally through a change of mindset in either party, so that the problem can be thought of in different ways, in a wider context, or with a new form of words. Instead of being a fixer or an adviser, the interviewer becomes a witness and questioner of the current story, and a proposer and collaborator for reframed stories. This way of looking at conversations puts both participants in a conversation on a more level field. It can absolve professionals from the sense of total responsibility for what happens – a sense of responsibility that so often oppresses them. A further advantage is that it removes the apparently pressing need to produce "endings" on each occasion. From a narrative point of view, no story really ever ends: it simply evolves.

Taking conversations seriously also means taking language and non-verbal communication seriously. It means making inquiry into the words that have actually been said, and the gestures accompanying them, and not into what one simply assumed the person meant – let alone into some quite extraneous matter that happens to have come into one's mind. This skill has often been likened to close reading in literary studies: a careful and precise attentiveness where one is able to notice nuances and ambiguities in what someone says. Rita Charon describes this as a shift from "listening like a doctor" to "listening like a reader" (Charon, 2016, p. 165). Much of the technical advice later in this book is concerned with how to develop and apply such attentiveness, in the form of careful questioning, or *narrative inquiry*.

Curiosity

Therapists often discuss what makes a professional encounter therapeutic. There is now a consensus that the common denominator here is a certain kind of curiosity (Cecchin, 1987). This is not intrusive curiosity. It is also entirely different from stereotypical or formulaic questioning. Instead, it means a focused and committed interest in where the story might go. Curiosity of this kind is not just something intellectual. It involves emotional engagement as well, so that there is an identification both with other people's feelings and with their own understanding of those feelings.

An essential part of therapeutic curiosity is a stance of *neutrality*. The term "neutrality," as used by family therapists, is not the same as of a lack of opinion, or of emotion, or of moral engagement. It is neutrality in the sense of being able to help clients with their own stories as they see them, and not as the interviewer necessarily expects them to be. It implies a tolerance of different points of view from one's own. It also demonstrates tolerance of several different points of view being expressed at different times, or by different individuals, including other family members (Palazzoli Selvini et al., 1980).

There is also a wider meaning to neutrality. It is neutrality in the face of all facts. This may take the form of setting aside a strong belief that someone's difficulties are mainly physical or, conversely, mainly psychological. It may even mean setting aside the notion that a problem exists – or indeed does not exist! The acid test will be whether the words and descriptions on offer are of utility to the other person. This expanded definition of neutrality has been defined as an intentional stance of "not knowing" (Anderson and Goolishian, 1992).

Learners often find the concept of neutrality hard to grasp, usually because they misunderstand it in a number of different ways. First, neutrality does *not* mean forgetting one's professional role with a recognised corpus of knowledge. Instead, it means recognising when, for a variety of reasons, this knowledge may not connect at all with the story of the other person in the room. Second, neutrality does not mean setting aside moral or legal standards and responsibility. It does not require practitioners to forsake their beliefs, nor the values that inspire their work. It certainly must not stop them from taking action in cases where someone's health or safety are significantly at risk. The aim of neutrality is not to disable action, but to pursue a fuller understanding of the problem. Third, it does not mean pretending that one can shed all the power – real or perceived – that comes with professional roles and affect conversations accordingly. Quite the contrary, it means holding it in mind constantly, taking account of it in one's utterances, and being transparent about it whenever possible.

Therapists sometimes quote the adage "The only person you can change is yourself." Remembering this is a good way to hold on to curiosity and a position of "not knowing." It invites professionals to be curious not only about their clients, but about themselves too: why they have become stuck, or determined to convince others of a particular truth, or annoyed if they cannot do so. It reminds professionals that they are unlikely to help others to develop a new story unless they have tried to appraise their own beliefs dispassionately in the conversation, to change their own story about what is going on.

The following case study demonstrates a GP applying curiosity. As nearly any professional will recognise, it also demonstrates the effectiveness of following the paradoxical advice "Don't just do something. Sit there!" One learner described it as "being liberated from the role of Dr Fixit."

Case example: a GP applies curiosity

Sam M is 35, divorced, and has been registered with me for five years. He first reported symptoms of excessive fatigue the year after he registered. The following year, he then had a bout of gastroenteritis that lasted for two weeks. Following this, he continued to have recurrent diarrhoea and abdominal pain. He also felt unwell and tired all the time. His tests at the hospital were all normal. As he was no better after two months, I referred him for a second opinion. The specialist made a diagnosis of "irritable bowel syndrome." Medication and a high-fibre diet produced little improvement in his symptoms. From September, he began to work from home for some of the time, although I did not learn about this until later. In March, he was reviewed by the specialist and started on an antidepressant. By April, he felt too unwell to work and requested a certificate to take time off work.

At this point, I felt I really needed to be more interested in him as a person. I started seeing him regularly and giving him longer to talk. He has a responsible and demanding job. He said he felt unable to return to work as he was still having unpredictable bouts of diarrhoea. I asked if he thought he would be able to get better if he did not have to return to work. It became apparent he was ambivalent in his feelings about his job. He described his boss as a "workaholic" and said he felt obliged to be the same, working long hours and weekends. As a result, he had lost friends and given up interests. Since he had been off work, his boss had been phoning frequently asking when he was returning.

I asked about his family, and he said he was close to his parents, who had been concerned for several years about his workload. He was previously married for a couple of years, and had no children. Since his marriage broke down, he hasn't been in a relationship and says he has just thrown himself into his work.

I've seen him three times now, for about 10 to 15 minutes each time. He has decided to resign from his present job, and when he is better look for a less stressful part-time job. He is planning a holiday with his brother. Since telling his boss he will not be returning, he has begun to feel better, with more energy and fewer bowel symptoms. He is still seeing me regularly, and I hope his physical symptoms will continue to improve now he has resolved his dilemma about his job. Mainly, what I have done is simply stay with his narrative, pick up words and phrases that engage my interests, and ask questions to help him expand on these.

Contexts

The patients and clients we see are surrounded by multiple contexts. Their stories have been constructed in conversations with families, friends, workmates or professionals they have seen previously. These in turn are embedded in history and geography, in lifelong personal and family experience, in gender and class relations, in interest groups and in faith communities. Understanding their narratives inevitably means inquiring into such contexts, including their family and work settings, and past encounters with professionals. It is often impossible to understand any utterance fully without an accurate understanding of its main contexts, and indeed the relationship between the various contexts (Pearce, 2007).

Practitioners bring their own contexts too. These include their training, traditions, regulations, professional codes of practice, and the organisational and societal cultures within which they work. They also include a wide range of personal contexts that may be very similar to the client's – or entirely different. When clients and practitioners converse, they are influenced by all sorts of professional contexts related to the work setting itself: booking systems, appointment lengths, the ways that the team operates, and so on. They are affected by their previous encounters, and by how well the participants already know each other. Patients do not talk to nurses in the same way they do to paramedics, care home managers or court officers. Nor do they talk to either of these in the way they talk to their greengrocers, bank managers, or their lovers. Every conversation we ever have is situated in a context, nesting within a set of other contexts.

One of the most important contexts for the patients and clients who see us is that our conversations with them are nearly always centred around perceived problems. For service users, this often means that they understandably place an emphasis on their difficulties rather than their resilience, in order to elicit care or entitlements. This in turn can put pressure on practitioners to offer certain automatic responses, either in the form of immediate acquiescence or by refusal. By contrast, a narrative-based approach involves seeing this "problem-oriented" context as an opportunity to carry out a more nuanced inquiry, and to see what kind of resolution might emerge from the conversation itself, rather than jumping to premature conclusions about whether a problem "deserves" a standard form of care or not.

When professional conversations fail, it is often because important contexts have not been noticed, or defined, or discussed. Many unsatisfactory or puzzling encounters can be freed up by talking about the professional and social contexts that surround them, or acknowledging the inevitable power relations that may be governing how others communicate with us: one description for this kind of transparency is "bringing the context into the room." Examples are limitless, but here are some examples of the kinds of questions we use to explore different contexts:

- "Before I can answer your question, it will help me to ask a few questions to understand what this all means to you . . . "
- "Since we've got only limited time, is there anything you think it's particularly important for me to concentrate on?"
- "Is there anything you're hoping I might say or do that's different from other professionals you've seen?"
- "You originally came from a different country. What do you think someone doing my job back home would say about this, or do about it?"
- "I'd be interested to know what you made of that experience as a black woman. Would you see racial discrimination as a possible factor, or is that not relevant here?"
- "Had you come today mainly hoping for reassurance, or was it something else?"
- "Who else do you think you might turn to for help with this problem?"
- "If we can't sort this problem out between the two of us, what do you think you might do next?"
- "Would it be OK if I just stay silent for a while and let you talk when you want?"

Complexity

Complexity conveys a view of the world as an infinite and unpredictable pattern of interactions. It means accepting that any narrative is only ever partial and provisional or – to use an analogy – like seeing one brief frame within a long and complicated video with a huge cast. This is a view that can be difficult for many health and social care professionals to take on board, because of our training in simple "linear" ideas such as formulations, labels, diagnoses, and the ideal treatment or solution. Yet in terms of work between professionals and others, and the story-making that goes on between them, complexity is an essential concept. It reminds us that the stories we participate in never truly stop, except insofar as we choose to punctuate them into encounters to suit our own pragmatic needs. It also reminds us that the stories made up between any two are the merest fraction of the stories that surround each of them, let alone the stories that surround those – and so on ad infinitum. Using complexity means aiming to move both interviewer and client away from fixed ideas of single causes and predictable effects, of unchangeable problems, and of over-concrete diagnoses and assessments. This can lead to stories that may be far more polyphonic, subtle, complex and interesting, and offer more potential for change, than the old ones.

How can complexity be brought into the everyday office meeting or home visit? The most important way is by continually following the other person's responses in the conversation, so that it effectively constitutes an extended set of "feedback loops" bringing wider perspectives into play. This depends on the use of what family therapists often call "circular questions" (Penn, 1983). The term "circular" is used not in the sense of "going round in circles," but to capture the idea of picking up what has just been said and opening this up with further questions. These may be questions that expand the view of the problem by inviting the patient to place it in a wider context of family relationships or time. They may be questions that literally circle around different family members present as an interviewer carefully poses questions in turn to explore how each person affects others in the family dance. They may in fact be any questions that reflect or transmit a view of the world functioning according to what have been called "complex responsive processes" (Stacey, 2001), where each person's spoken contributions impact on others around them, in an endless chain of influence. These and other kinds of questions are discussed in greater detail in the next chapter.

Case example: a mental health social worker explores complexity in someone's story

I visited a patient who was about to be discharged from a mental hospital following an episode of severe depression. She had a facial deformity following a car accident, and this had triggered her depression. When I saw her, I was quite shocked at the disfigurement. We talked about the way other people in her life were reacting to her appearance.

I started to ask her some questions about this: who, in her family, was most worried about her condition? She replied without hesitation that it was her father, who is widowed and lives back in Italy. I asked her some more questions: what did this mean to herself, and to the other important people in her life? She explained that she was the only child. There was hefty pressure on her to go back and live with her father and look after him, which would have been "the done thing" in Italian families, where an unmarried daughter was expected to care for parents for the full duration of their lives. Her family were counselling her against getting any further surgery on her face, and in her mind this was connected with their wish for her to be "a proper daughter" and look after her father as her first priority.

Using questions in this way, I learned a great deal about her family's inter-actions, as well as beliefs about what had happened to her. This helped her to look at her own confusion as to whether she wished to care for her fam-ily, or whether she wished her family to care for her, as she had now suffered a deformity. She told me that she had enormous difficulty in getting on with her father, and could not contemplate living with him. She also felt guilty, as she had pursued a career that evoked disapproval from the whole family.

I remember this conversation because I was struck how this kind of ques-tioning gave me an additional resource at my disposal. It helped me and my patient to look at the far wider implications of what had happened to her, and her depression. It was also such a strong feeling of "bringing an entire family into the room," even though only a single member was with me.

Challenge

There is a difference between just being an attentive listener – itself an essential and important skill – and being able to question someone's story in a way that offers the potential for new and unexpected directions. As emphasised previously, this does not involve "nudging" clients in the direction that you hope they might go, let alone firmly directing them to do so (unless the circumstances carry signifi-cant risk). Instead, effective challenge involves inviting people to consider their concerns from new and possibly original perspectives.

Closely linked with the idea of challenge is that of *creativity* – so much so that some of our trainers prefer to use this word in its place. A narrative approach sees conversations as a process in which two or more individuals are continually inter-weaving their original stories so that they can jointly create a new one. In a health or social care setting, the roles of the two participants in the act of creation are not the same. The patient brings a problem and the professional is paid to help with it. The latter therefore has a dual role – both as a participant and as someone who has to monitor and assist in the progress of the new story. One useful way to frame this dual role is to see the professional as an "observer-participant" in the act of narrative reconstruction. The observer function depends on attentiveness and respect towards narrators and their existing stories. The participant function involves an awareness that almost any story has the capacity to move in new and more helpful directions, especially if this is done through careful questions, and these are incremental and unprejudiced. It means neither accepting an account naively as an unassailable account of the truth, nor rejecting it as fabricated, but instead looking out for opportunities to ask how it might evolve if seen in a different light.

Caution

It requires sensitivity to monitor one's own emotional responses, and to make sure one is matching the questions to suit others and their capacity to extend their thinking at that moment. Many learners report that they sense if they are pushing the level of challenge too far by monitoring their own level of anxiety, or what is happening in their own bodies – for example, by noticing muscle tension in their faces or stomachs. They then know to pull back and make the conversation more friendly and affirming until a more appropriate opportunity arises to offer challenge. Some interviewers do this intuitively. Our experience is that most can learn to do so.

Learners who become fired by narrative ideas can become excessively challenging. They can bombard others with questions when they do not want to talk, or just want advice. They can also start to behave as if they were formal therapists. This is inappropriate. Service users usually do not come to health and social care for pure therapy, and can find it alienating. Besides, the time is almost always too short for this, and the social setting quite inappropriate. Although many learners do go through an unsettling period when they are adapting to a new way of seeing their work (and sometimes their world), it will usually not help them if they devalue or abandon everything they have learned before. The most inspired learners are often those who have been able to make their own synthesis – their own new professional narrative – by incorporating a number of different approaches into a narrative framework. The next case example is an account of a "Conversation Inviting Change" that quite simply went wrong.

Case example: a physiotherapist misjudges a conversation

A 25-year-old man, Andrew H, came to see me about pains in his shoulders. He explained he had been lifting furniture. It seemed likely that his shoulder pain was a trivial strain, and I found myself far more interested in his look of distress. I asked him why he had been lifting furniture. He told me that he had just left his first job as he could not cope with the stress any more, and moved back with his mother. I invited him back for another appointment, not so much because I thought he needed more treatment, but because I wanted to give him a chance to talk more.

He duly returned for another appointment, and while I was treating him I found out about his family. He was the youngest child, but his parents had divorced. The father had not kept in touch with the family. He had always felt that his mother didn't like him, perhaps because he was born when the marriage was already failing, and left him out of things, favouring the three siblings. Now back in the family home having failed to stay away, he felt that his mother thought worse of him than ever. His mother was not in touch with her own parents who were in Scotland, as Andrew thought his father was too.

At the end of the appointment, I felt that I had understood much more about Andrew and his problems. However, I noticed that he looked miserable, and I asked how he had found the family discussion. He replied, "I think you are wasting my time – I don't want to talk about my family. It isn't why I came." I felt disconcerted by this.

This case helped me to understand the importance of setting the context for dialogue outside the usual expectations of a meeting with a physio. I had used my power to intrude into personal areas that the patient might rather keep private. Since this experience, I have tried to offer a discussion of family background to a patient as an option of potential interest and use to both of us, just as a physical investigation like an X-ray might be.

Care

As an approach, "Conversations Inviting Change" is aimed to help others, and above all to care for them. It is not a purely cognitive approach, designed to engage only with someone's logical thinking, but rooted instead in compassion and practical ethics. None of the "C's" will work in the way intended unless the person applying them is careful, attentive and kind. When this is not the case, for whatever reason, we counsel that the interviewer should try in the first instance to reflect on why this is occurring (including a clash of beliefs with the client, or through the pressures of everyday work), and remedy this where possible. This may mean postponing the rest of the conversation for another date – or discussing this with a neutral colleague in order to achieve greater detachment from whatever is interfering with the duty of care. It may even mean abandoning any attempt to apply "Conversations Inviting Change" with that person, especially if they are expecting a more conventional approach from a practitioner and are patently disconcerted by anything else.

Finally, we have changed our own list of "C's" over the years since Caroline Lindsey first devised the original ones, in response to feedback from learners. In the original edition of this book, there were only "six C's," and these included "co-creation," which was dropped as some regarded it as jargon, and "circularity," which is now covered as part of the guidance on questioning (see the next chapter). Indeed, readers may want to consider which of the above "seven C's" they find more or less useful, which further "C's" they might wish to add, or even to compile a list that fits their own understanding of what it means to be a caring and effective practitioner, applying their own most valued principles.

Box 2.1   Conversations inviting change: the "seven C's" in summary

Conversations. Effective conversations don't just describe reality, they create new understanding of it. Conversations can be seen as interventions in their own right: the end as well as the means. Simply by taking place, they create opportunities for people to rethink and redefine their realities.

Curiosity. This is what turns conversations from chatter into something more substantial. It invites others to reframe their stories in different ways. An essential aspect of curiosity is aspiring to neutrality (to individuals, to blame, to interpretations, to facts). Curiosity should also extend to yourself. What are your own thoughts about the interaction? How can you become curious about your own biases and prejudices, or prevent yourself being critical or impatient? How does your role or power limit the kind of neutrality you can offer?

Contexts. This is what it is most effective to be curious about. Important contexts in work with patients and clients are families, cultures, beliefs and faith. In conversations between practitioners, they include teams, organisations and professional networks, hierarchies, history, geography, and belief systems and values.

Complexity. Rather than looking for a "quick fix" in every situation, it is better to consider any problem as part of an infinite and unpredicatable dance of interactions. A sense of complexity gets away from fixed ideas of cause and effect, unchangeable problems, and over-concrete solutions. Instead, it emphasises ideas such as emergence, evolution and gradual resolution.

Challenge. Professional conversations can be seen as a form of shared activity, in which one person is challenging another to think of a different description of what is going on. What you are looking for is a better account of reality than the present one, which means a way of narrating the story that makes better sense for others of what they are going through, and may include practical actions.

Caution. You need to use sensitivity, and monitor your own emotional responses, to make sure you are matching your words to suit the other person and their capacity to extend their thinking at that moment. If someone wants straightforward information and advice, be prepared to give it (while being aware of the limitations of doing so without an opportunity for the other person to make sense of it for themselves). Also, remember you're not doing therapy – on colleagues or on patients!

Care. The role of health and social care professionals is to look after others. None of the ideas and techniques will work unless you are respectful, affectionate and attentive. Narrative-based practice needs to be grounded in moral commitment.

Suggested exercises

1 Review an encounter with a client or patient. What contexts did you inquire into? What other contexts might you ask about on another occasion?

2 How far was the final story constructed with the patient? Are there things you could have said or asked to make it collaborative?

3 Choose one of the "seven C's." Think about it during an encounter (or take each concept in turn, one per encounter.) How well does the concept fit what is going on in the conversation? Does it suggest any new ways of saying things or of asking questions?

4 When time is not too pressing, try to observe your own chain of questioning with a client. How far is it led by habit and how far does it follow his or her language?

5 After an encounter, jot down some questions you would like to ask the client or patient the next time.

6 Are there additional "C's" you would add to your personal list? Or could you make a similar list using another letter? Or in your own first language if it is not English?

References

Anderson, H. and Goolishian, H. (1992) The client is the expert: a not-knowing approach to therapy. In S. McNamee and K. Gergen (eds), *Therapy as Social Construction*. London: Sage, pp. 25–39.

Cecchin, G. (1987) Hypothesising, circularity, and neutrality revisited: an invitation to curiosity. *Family Process*, 26, 405–413.

Charon, R. (2016) Close reading: the signature method of narrative medicine. In R. Charon, S. DasGupta, N. Hermann, C. Irvine, E.R. Marcus, E. Riviera Colòn, et al. (eds), *The Principles and Practice of Narrative Medicine*. Oxford: Oxford University Press, pp. 157–179.

Palazzoli Selvini, M., Boscolo, L., Cecchin, G. and Prata, G. (1980) Hypothesising-circularity-neutrality: three guidelines for the conductor of the session. *Family Process*, 19, 3–12.

Pearce, W.B. (2007) *Making Social Worlds: A Communications Perspective*. Oxford: Wiley-Blackwell.

Penn, P. (1983) Circular questioning. *Family Process*, 21, 267–280.

Stacey, R. (2001) *Complex Responsive Processes in Organisations: Learning and Knowledge Creation*. Abingdon: Routledge.

CHAPTER THREE

Narrative inquiry

Key ideas in this chapter

- A crucial skill in narrative-based practice is that of narrative inquiry: an ability to ask precise and carefully focused questions.
- Effective questions arise from hypotheses about what it might be useful to discuss, including causes, reasons and explanations for what the other person is speaking about.
- They also depend on responsiveness to feedback (circularity), and maintaining a stance of neutrality.
- There are some formal ways of categorising types of questions, and these can be useful when learning to do good questioning. However, nothing can substitute for spontaneous inquiry that exactly fits the person, the story and the moment.

Introduction

This chapter is devoted to the art of narrative inquiry. The guidance below describes what we think is effective practice in this respect. It draws principally on the ideas of a group of Italian psychiatrists known as the Milan Team (Palazzoli Selvini et al., 1980; Cecchin, 1987; Tomm, 1988). Although they did not call themselves narrative practitioners, they were very influential in encouraging family therapists to take the non-interpretive stance that most use nowadays. The principles they described are probably the most helpful ones for creating a narrative-based stance.

Learners often ask us to provide lists of "good questions." Although we sometimes respond by offering generic question stems that may prove useful (and some are listed below), on the whole we prefer to ask people to note the questions they have found useful from their own work and experience, and consider why these worked. As always, everything depends on the context. In general, it is probably more useful to think of good *questioning* rather than good questions. A question that is brilliant in one conversation may fall flat or be hopelessly off target in another conversation. In the same way, a question that worked well at one moment in a dialogue might have had a negative effect if the timing had been different, the tone of voice wrong, or the emotions fabricated. Inevitably, there are circumstances where questioning may in fact be entirely inappropriate or need to be very restricted, or when silence is preferable.

Why are questions necessary?

The purpose of narrative inquiry is not to persuade someone to see things your way, or to solve problems for them. It is to create opportunities for people to think about their stories in new ways. The views people reach, and any actions that result, may be quite different from anything that you expected or hoped for. Often, the change that occurs in the conversation is a simply a shift in thinking, rather than a concrete decision. For example, someone may realise in the course of a conversation that what they were already thinking or doing was right all along, and feel more comfortable about it. Alternatively, they may reach an entirely different view of the problem, sometimes at variance from your own. This in turn may necessitate a transparent discussion of why these differences have arisen, what the extent of negotiability may be on either side, and how they might be resolved.

Good questioning is often (although not always) a better way of creating openness and possibility in conversation than other forms of speech. Good questioners can demonstrate how well they have understood a client simply by pursuing their inquiry in a way that corresponds appropriately to the language and the emotions present in the conversation. Unlike some other schools of thought, when we teach "Conversations Inviting Change," we discourage empathic noises and comments (e.g. "I hear what you're saying"), reflection (e.g. "So what you're saying is . . . "), reformulation (e.g. "It sounds to me as if . . . "), and interpretation (e.g. "I think what's really going on here is . . . "). Although there is sometimes a place for these kinds of utterances, as a way of showing interest and understanding, good questioning can generally demonstrate this even more – with the added benefit of introducing further movement into the conversation.

For the same reason, and also in contrast to some counselling approaches, we try to discourage direct inquiry into emotions (including the ubiquitous "How did you feel about that?"). For some clinicians, this technique has become an automatic response, asked without sincerity, and sometimes inappropriately. Similarly, while a statement such as "You must have felt very angry" may be said with the intention of expressing empathy, it might be experienced as clumsy – and may be off the mark anyway. If someone is feeling strong emotion and wants to express it, a question such as "How did this affect you?" will allow them to do so. Essentially, we promote the use of any questions or utterances that open space for expansion of the narrative, rather than closing it down by expressing preconceived ideas. It is a useful discipline to avoid questions beginning with a verb (e.g. "Do you?" or "Can you?"), which may lead to short and uninformative answers. By contrast, if you make a habit of using words such as "what," "how" or "when," these will usually bring out fuller and more helpful answers.

The Milan Team proposed three guidelines or principles for effective inquiry (or what they termed "interviewing"): *hypothesising, circularity* and *neutrality*. Later, one of the team, Gianfranco Cecchin, proposed a fourth principle: *curiosity*. The sections that follow examine each of these principles in turn. Following the usage of the Milan Team, the term "interviewer" is sometimes used here to mean the person conducting narrative inquiry.

Hypothesising

When they talked about hypothesising, the Milan Team were drawing attention to the fact that it is almost impossible *not* to form ideas in your mind about the purpose of the conversation, along with the causes, reasons, explanations and interpretations for anything the other person says. However, there are two quite different ways of responding to your own ideas. On the one hand, you can assume that everything you think is correct and helpful, simply because you have thought of it, and try to persuade the other person this is the case. On the other hand, you can regard your own ideas just as different possible descriptions of what is going on, and to try to establish through inquiry whether these descriptions are of any interest or use to the other person, or will help to progress matters. This involves the discipline of becoming sceptical about your own ideas, restrained about imposing them, and thus formulating a question that gives no hint of your opinion. It also involves being able to let go of an idea immediately if it turns out not to be useful to the other person.

Some learners report that they are rarely conscious of their hypotheses, or only fleetingly so, but feel that they are still able to question clients effectively through intuition alone. Where this is the case, the process may be happening at a non-conscious level. More often, however, we observe that questioners who are unaware of their hypotheses may pursue a whole line of inquiry based on a single unexamined assumption – perhaps related to their own experience. Some people call this "being wedded to your hypothesis." When a professional conversation appears to be stuck, it is always worth trying to find out whether an unwarranted assumption of any kind is present, and adapting one's input accordingly.

Constant calibration with the client's narrative through careful questioning is the most reliable way of avoiding misplaced assumptions. In Box 3.1, the two conversations from the beginning of Chapter 1 appear again, but this time with the likely underlying hypotheses identified in square brackets.

Box 3.1 Occupational therapists carrying out the same task in different ways [with hypotheses shown]

Therapist A (taking a normative approach)

Therapist A:	Well, as you know, I've come to look at your home because of your falls. [Hypothesis: I am here to prevent this client's falls.]
Client:	I've had a lot of them lately.
Therapist A:	Yes, your social worker mentioned that. So let's go round and look at what we can do for you. [Hypothesis: The client agrees that she wants me to prevent her falls. She doesn't seem very talkative anyway.]

Therapist B (using a narrative-based stance)

Therapist B:	Well, as you know, I've come to look at your home because of your falls. [Hypothesis: I've come here to have a conversation about falls, but I need to know more before taking any action.]
Client:	Yes, I've had a lot of them lately.
Therapist B:	Did anything cause this, do you think? [Hypothesis: The client may have some ideas about the causes of the falls. If I try to draw her out, it may help me understand more.]
Client:	Oh, I thought the social worker would have told you. My son used to live here and always helped me get around.
Therapist B:	Is he not here any more? [Hypothesis: The son's absence sounds significant and I need to know more.]
Patient:	No, that's the terrible thing. He got killed in a car accident . . .

Readers may want to revisit some of the other conversations in Chapter 1, identifying possible hypotheses that informed the questioning.

Circularity

The Milan Team's guideline of circularity covers the idea that the person carrying out the inquiry (whether in a consultation, supervision or some other professional context) should always note in careful detail what the response is to each question, and use this to frame what follows. This involves a willingness to "go with the flow" of a conversation, even if this is moving in a quite different direction from the expected one. This in turn implies an ability to respond with equal interest, whether or not the ideas in one's own mind are confirmed. Whenever possible, it is worthwhile for interviewers to pick up on words or phrases from the other person's own narrative rather than choosing from their own vocabulary, or substituting other words and phrases that may seem almost identical but may have significant differences for someone else.

The activity of asking questions is one that comes naturally to people who work in health and social care – and fits with the expectations of patients and clients as well. That is a significant advantage. It distinguishes them, for example, from counsellors and psychotherapists, who often use other kinds of utterances, such as offering interpretations ("I think your symptoms are an expression of unresolved grief"), using encouraging phrases ("go on," "tell me more"), or simply reflecting back what the person has just said. It is also helpful that people coming to health and social care settings expect to be asked questions and are generally prepared to give answers. In many ways, therefore, the clinic, office or home setting is already set up for the process of narrative inquiry.

However, the questions that form part of narrative inquiry are generally quite different from traditional forms of professional conversation. The principal difference is that professionals traditionally use questioning to narrow down possibilities, whereas narrative inquiry is aimed at opening them up. This is not in order to have a longer encounter, but in order to use time in the most efficient way, by seeking exactly the words and contexts that are most important to pursue. Some practitioners have an ability to sense cues, words that have "life" or "weight" in them, and to tune out of everything superfluous. Others seem to pick words at random from the client's flow and hence ask questions that are irrelevant or trivial. One corrective to this is to check constantly which among several possible cues it might be most helpful for the practitioner to follow. This may involve reviewing the conversation or winding it backwards whenever a question seems to lead down a blind alley or makes the interview go slack (e.g. "You mentioned earlier that there were two aspects to this problem: which of them is foremost in your mind at the moment?"). Another approach is to ask the other person how the conversation is going for them, what they are getting out of it, and what is still missing for them (e.g. "How are we doing so far in the conversation, in relation to the issue you brought?"). This offers clients the possibility of re-setting the agenda as they see fit.

With good conversations, there is a circularity of emotions as well as words. Some poor interviewers meander from one question to the next, with no apparent connecting thread, while others, conversely, go straight for the jugular vein. Effective practitioners seem to move forward at exactly the right pace to keep the conversation taut without provoking either boredom or defensiveness. When a client seems vague or unfocused, they become more precise in their questioning. When a client tenses up and there is a sense that they have run up against a "wall" in the conversation, the interviewer eases up gently but not too much (or alternatively, pauses to ask "How is this conversation going for you?").

The process of hypothesising and circularity is illustrated in Figure 3.1, starting at the top.

An example of this process at work during a conversation appears in Box 3.2.

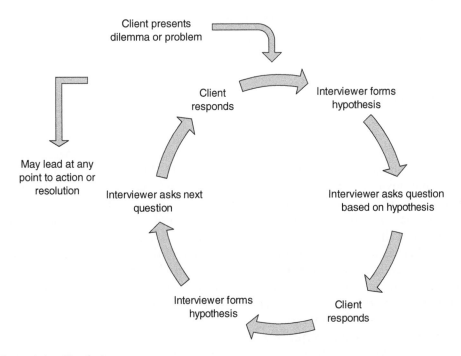

Figure 3.1 Circularity

Box 3.2 **An interviewer forms hypotheses and frames questions in response to a client's narrative**

Client:	I'm not sure whether to tell my husband I've spent so much.
Interviewer:	[silently forming a hypothesis that the client may be scared of doing so] What would stop you doing so?
Client:	[after reflecting whether to disclose this] He sometimes flies off the handle when I do.
Interviewer:	[after considering how to help client develop her narrative] Can you give me an example of when this happened?
Client:	Well, there was this relatively minor incident . . . [gives example of when her husband shouted at her].
Interviewer:	[forming a new hypothesis that there may have been major incidents as well as "minor" ones] What's it like when incidents aren't so minor?
Client:	[begins to disclose more serious incidents involving physical harm, leading to discussion of sources of help and protection].

Our experience is that these kinds of carefully calibrated exchanges, tailored to the exact words clients use, are more likely to nurture trust, and therefore to lead to fuller narratives.

Neutrality

The Milan Team's third guideline – neutrality – flows from the previous two. As discussed in the previous chapter, it expresses the idea that interviewers should constantly maintain an open, tolerant stance that allows the other person the maximum possible space, unimpeded by the intrusive beliefs or prejudices of the interviewer. The Milan Team were at pains to emphasise that this did *not* mean that interviewers should have no beliefs and prejudices of their own. Nor did they ever rule out the possibility of situations (including dangerous or life-threatening ones), where it was legitimate and ethical to declare these. What they did argue, however, was that clinicians very often found themselves in situations where they could do more harm by inappropriate certainty than by carefully considered neutrality. It is therefore preferable in general to follow the discipline of not *showing* views or opinions to clients.

For some learners, it may not be easy to master the process of turning a hypothesis (whether conscious or intuitive) into a neutral question, and making sure it does not give everything away by its wording or intonation, or alternatively seem bland and disengaged. That is one of the reasons for using structured training methods in small groups – including the use of pauses to give interviewers time to consider their hypotheses and turn these into genuinely open and neutral questions. With practice, the process becomes internalised and hence easier. For some people, it fits so well with what they believe to be effective and ethical conversational practice that it becomes effortless.

There are clearly encounters where it is impossible to sustain neutral questioning throughout a whole conversation. On some occasions, the interviewer may have professional duties that need to be followed, regardless of the client's wishes. Obvious examples include the times when social workers need to break the news of a statutory procedure, or doctors have to refuse to sign statements requested on inadequate grounds. Interviewers can certainly use neutral questioning in the opening part of such conversations, in order to establish the other person's view and what they are expecting. However, at some point, they will need to declare their position and conduct the rest of the conversation on the explicit basis that they have the authority to override the other person's wishes. Even then, it may still be possible to use neutral questioning to explore the effect of the decision. If such exchanges cannot be conducted in a strictly neutral way, there is often no reason why they cannot be civil, respectful and transparent: "I realise this wasn't what you were hoping for. Where is this decision going to leave you?" This kind of scenario is addressed further in Chapter 5, under the heading of managing disagreement and hostility.

Curiosity

One member of the Milan Team, Gianfranco Cecchin (1987), wrote a further paper where he boiled down the approach of the team into one word: "curiosity." He suggested that if an interviewer felt and expressed adequate curiosity, everything else would follow automatically. This would include not only a helpful exploration of the nature and content of the problem, but also the response to the interview itself. "How helpful are you finding this conversation? Are there any other questions I should have asked you? Am I getting the balance of questions to advice about right? Am I showing any prejudices that are getting in the way of your thinking?" On our courses, people receiving supervision from their peers during group work often report that it was not any specific inquiry that helped in a conversation (at least so far as they can remember), but the overall stance of curiosity in their interviewer. Indeed, we have sometimes seen quite clunky questions do the trick so long as the person carrying out the interview was genuinely engaged and curious. Conversely, an inquiry that appears to be technically perfect may achieve nothing at all, if delivered in a way that seems rehearsed or inauthentic.

There may be a few specific questions in any interview that stop people in their tracks and lead them to say "That's a really good question." There may be others that they chew over during the course of the following week so that the interviewer may never even learn how good a question it was. Many of us have also had the humbling experience of being congratulated by someone after an interview for asking fantastic questions that we never actually asked. Clients have simply imagined that they heard what that they really wanted to be asked, or formulated this in their own minds. In these instances, it was the interviewer's attitude itself that had most effect: one of engaged curiosity.

Interventive interviewing

The principles of the Milan Team were subsequently developed into a framework for questioning by Karl Tomm, a Canadian professor of psychiatry. He called it "interventive interviewing." He chose the term to indicate that conversations conducted mainly through inquiry can make a difference to how people view and understand things. We have always preferred to use the gentler-sounding term "Conversations Inviting Change," but are essentially describing the same process (Tomm, 1988).

Tomm divided questions into four categories: lineal, circular, strategic and reflexive. As he pointed out, this taxonomy does not map very well onto many real-life conversations. Our own observation is that it can also hamper people if they try to follow it slavishly. Like riding a bike, it is probably best learned and then forgotten. However, some learners find it useful to know the distinctions in order to monitor their own technique in the early stages of trying out narrative inquiry.

Lineal questions

Tomm called his first category of questions "lineal" ones (some learners prefer to use the more familiar word "linear" to describe them). Such questions allow interviewers to ascertain the facts orient themselves in the important contexts, and gain a clearer understanding of the other person's story.

Some examples:

- "What has happened?"
- "How long has this been an issue for you?"
- "Who else is involved?"
- "Who else believes . . . ?"
- "What have you done about . . . ?"

Although lineal questions bring out useful factual and contextual information, they carry the drawback of tending to establish and even consolidate the existing story, rather than help the other person to see new paths or options. They also need to be used with caution because they can unintentionally convey an inquisitorial or judgemental attitude.

Circular questions

As described in the previous chapter, circular questions are any that evoke a view of matters as complex and non-linear. They can also be thought of as "interactional" questions. They assume that everything in life is somehow connected with everything else, in a pattern of interacting loops. Circular questions are used to bring out patterns that link together events, perceptions and behaviour, or differentiate these.

Some examples:

- "How do you think x sees you?"
- "How do you imagine x thinks you see her?"
- "When x gets angry, what does y do?"
- "When the consultant/senior partner is stressed, what effect does that have on the receptionists?"
- "Was the nurse more likely to show this attitude problem before or after her colleague went on sick leave?"

Some of the questions used by professionals when applying conventional methods of conversation also happen to be circular questions. All those familiar litanies ("How long? Where? What makes you feel worse?") can therefore provide an easy entry into creating a much broader-ranging narrative ("When was the worst time ever? What was your understanding of why it happened at that time? When do you get fears it might return as badly?"). This makes it possible to ask effective circular questions, and still carry out a routine professional task.

Strategic questions

These are questions where the interviewer intentionally embeds advice in the question. This can be helpful when a practitioner genuinely needs to act as an advisor or instructor but wishes to modulate their stance in doing so. Offering suggestions in the form of a question certainly leaves more room for the other person to reflect on their response than if they received direct advice. With the right tone of voice and in the right circumstances, this can also be experienced as reassuring and supportive. They can also come over as too directive, however well-intentioned they might be, and should therefore be used sparingly.

Some examples:

- "What do you think would happen if you . . .
  - started a disciplinary procedure?"
  - just ignored this?"
  - spoke to your partner/boss about this?"
  - got legal advice?"

- "What would the advantages and disadvantages be if you . . .
  - said exactly what you think?"
  - asked x to do y?"
  - just told her what to do?"
  - asked what she would like?"
  - pointed out what it says in her contract about this?"

Reflexive questions

Reflexive questions are ones that invite people to consider familiar issues in unfamiliar contexts, or from a new perspective. Hence, their effect is to induce reflexivity – an observer perspective on oneself – in the person being questioned. These are the questions that often seem to "stop people in their tracks." Although they can be experienced as challenging, reflexive questions offer a more creative approach than other types of questioning.

Some examples:

- "What will happen if nothing changes?"/"How long do you think you could put up with the situation if it doesn't change?"
- "What would happen if you do nothing?"/"Who else do you think would be the first to act if you did nothing yourself?"
- "What is the best/worst thing that could happen?"
- "If the team couldn't resolve their disagreements, who do you think would be the first person to leave?"
- "If we could find a solution to this problem, what other problems might be exposed as a result?"
- "What can we do to move this conversation forward?"
- "What would you do if this happened again?"

From these examples, it should be clear that the same question may fit into different categories depending on why and how it is asked. There may also be a difference between the interviewer's intention in asking a question and the actual effects on the interviewee. Practitioners need to be aware that no question can ever be entirely neutral. Simply by being asked, it will focus the conversation on a particular area that the professional has chosen, which may or may not chime with the other person's interests and preoccupations. In that broader sense, every question is "strategic." Once again, the responsibility lies with the practitioner to sustain an awareness of why particular questions have or have not been used, and the effect they are having.

Solution-focused questions

Another approach to questions that has been used within family therapy, and that we have adopted to some extent into "Conversations Inviting Change," is drawn from a school of thought known as solution-focused therapy (De Shazer, 1985). The approach is based on assuming that change is always possible, that professional conversations should be focused on exceptions to problems rather than the problems themselves, and should be directed towards achievable goals. Typical forms of questioning include the following (Greene and Lee, 2011):

- The miracle question: "If there was a miracle overnight, how would you know it had happened?"
- The time machine question: "If you could travel into the future when the problem was solved, what would be better for you?"
- The outcome question: "If I met you in the street three months after our meetings finished, what would I notice was different about you?"
- Relationship question: "Who would be the first person to notice things were different, and what would they see?"

Although this approach can occasionally be used in everyday encounters in health and social care, this needs to be sparing and integrated into more natural forms of interchange in order to avoid creating the impression of using a "box of tricks."

Michael White and "externalising" questions

The Australian family therapist Michael White, whose work was discussed in the Introduction, is known for a particular approach to narrative inquiry based on the idea of "externalisation" (White, 2007). This involves seeing any problem as having an existence that is independent of any particular person, and as if, metaphorically speaking, it has a life of its own. Examples include the following (adapted from Parton and O'Byrne, 2000; Roscoe et al., 2011):

- "How does this problem try to intimidate you?"
- "When aggression holds you hostage like this, what do you find are the best ways to escape?"
- "What has guilt tried to talk you into doing?"
- "How has the fear tried to convince you that it's unsafe to go out?"
- "What are the ways that the worry stops you from doing things?"

In the context of formal therapy, or extended therapeutic work carried out by fully trained practitioners, it can be helpful to use ideas and language such as this. It can engage an individual or family, and help them gain control over the difficulties that appeared to possess them. Our experience in teaching narrative-based practice to professionals working in more everyday circumstances and with limited amounts of time is that these kinds of questions can also seem too distant from everyday discourse. At the same time, an understanding of the principles of externalisation can help practitioners become aware of the tremendous power of metaphor, and its potential use in enhancing people's sense of agency and control over their lives.

In our training courses, we have used the ideas of the Milan Team, Tomm, solution-focused therapists and Michael White in all sorts of ways, but have put most stress on what characterises narrative inquiry overall: attentiveness to language and gesture, and on following feedback responsively. From our observations, most health and social care professionals are quite empathic and sensitive to the general tone of feeling in a conversation, but they may have inadequate skills in noticing the tiny giveaway words, phrases and physical movements that can act as cues for curiosity and focused questioning. Training in narrative inquiry allows them to become more attuned to others, and enhances their ability to calibrate their verbal and non-verbal interventions accordingly from moment to moment.

Suggested exercises

1 Try to jot down some of the questions you ask in a professional encounter. Afterwards, consider what the hypotheses may have been underlying these questions.
2 Reviewing these or other questions you asked in an encounter, consider whether these conveyed a genuinely curious and neutral stance, or whether you might have expressed them in a way that did this more.

3   Make a record of questions you ask that appear to stop people in their tracks and consider their difficulties or dilemmas from a new perspective. What do you think are the most effective questions you have ever asked in a professional setting?

References

Cecchin, G. (1987) Hypothesising, circularity, and neutrality revisited: an invitation to curiosity. *Family Process*, 26, 405–413.

De Shazer, S. (1985) *Keys to Solution in Brief Therapy*. New York: Norton.

Greene, G.J. and Lee, M.Y. (2011) *Solution-Oriented Social Work Practice: An Integrative Approach to Working with Client Strengths*. Oxford: Oxford University Press.

Palazzoli Selvini, M., Boscolo, L., Cecchin, G. and Prata, G. (1980) Hypothesising-circularity-neutrality: three guidelines for the conductor of the session. *Family Process*, 19, 3–12.

Parton, N. and O'Byrne, P. (2000) *Constructive Social Work: Towards a New Practice*. Basingstoke: Macmillan.

Roscoe, K.D., Carson, A.M. and Madoc-Jones, L. (2011). Narrative social work: conversations between theory and practice. *Journal of Social Work Practice*, 25(1), 47–61.

Tomm, K. (1988) Interventive interviewing: part III. Intending to ask lineal, circular, strategic or reflexive questions? *Family Process*, 27(1), 1–15.

White, M. (2007) *Maps of Narrative Practice*. New York: Norton.

CHAPTER FOUR

What hinders narratives

Key ideas in this chapter

- Nearly every practitioner reports having to work under increasing pressure, with less time for patients and clients, with the presence of computers making meaningful conversations harder.
- Many also feel that the dominance of guidelines and protocols makes them unconfident or unwilling to offer more person-centred or creative consultations.
- Many practitioners report being aware of displaying habits that inhibit their clients from developing helpful narratives.
- Many also appear to have a preference for targeting strong emotions or seeking psychological explanations without realising that this can also impair narratives.
- It is possible to become more aware of common obstacles to narrative development and to finds ways of avoiding these.

Introduction

Many health and social professionals report that the environments in which they work make it hard to adopt narrative-based practice. Typical constraints include reduced time for each encounter, the imperative to record consultations meticulously, the distracting presence of computers, and the need to follow protocols or guidelines. In many work settings, these challenges are compounded by the large proportion of their patients or clients who may not have English as their first language, and hence may need others to interpret for them. Reduced continuity of care, and the introduction of new ways of working, including telehealth and phone consultations, may also lessen opportunities to conduct more leisurely or reflective encounters.

Such external pressures can lead practitioners to behave and speak in stereotypical ways that are mainly aimed at getting tasks done and increasing perceived "productivity." In addition, some of the interviewing styles that are widely taught may paradoxically add to the problem, by encouraging automatic ways of interacting that appear superficially to be "person-centred" but in practice are applied somewhat formulaically, or fail to allow enough flexibility for each individual or from moment to moment. This chapter examines some common hindrances to narrative flow, and offers guidance about how to overcome these. The next chapter complements this guidance with specific hints and tips about how to help narratives develop.

The following examples demonstrate the kinds of hindrances that practitioners have reported, or that we have observed in videos, role play or training exercises. What they all share is that the interviewer in each instance is offering a response that is at odds to a greater or lesser extent with the ideas and language that are actually emerging in the conversation. These examples are fictional ones, compiled for training purposes only. They are each followed by suggestions of how to avoid or overcome the particular pitfall illustrated.

Being dominated by time

Practitioner: What's brought you here today?
Client: Well, I've had a letter from the council that I'm quite worried about.
Practitioner: OK, let me have a look at it [taking it from the client's hand].

Exchanges such as this happen a lot. They seem to be based on the idea that cutting corners will save time. In reality, the opposite may be the case. A minute or two of inquiry to establish the context may save a great deal of time later, for example by making sure the professional doesn't get drawn straight into an erroneous set of assumptions. Simply asking "Can you give me a bit of background?" or "What has made you concerned?" might pre-empt this.

Being dominated by the records

Client: I had an accident a few weeks ago and I've been seeing one of your colleagues about what happened.
Practitioner: Fine. Let me just check the notes and see what my colleague has written.

There is often an assumption that a client's previous records will contain a more accurate or official version of the truth than the narrative they are currently bringing.

This may of course be untrue even at the factual level, since the records may be incomplete or incorrect. Even when that is not the case, disqualifying the client's narrative in this way may leave them feeling patronised and disempowered. Allowing them to retell the story can overcome both of these risks ("Yes, I've seen your notes, but do you mind telling me briefly what happened . . . ?").

Imposing the professional agenda

Client: I've really just come to collect the form. I'm doing fine generally.
Practitioner: Yes. I see that we haven't done an overall review recently . . .

There is nothing wrong with following good evidence-based practice by carrying out regular reviews or whatever routines the professional is required to undertake. The failure here, however, is one of contextualisation. The interviewer misses a cue for congratulating the person on being fine, and ignores the possible implication that he or she might prefer on this occasion just walking off with the appropriate form. There are no doubt many occasions when professionals need to be able to convey the message "I can see that you want to leave, but I need to check something else before you do." The problem is that many practitioners report that they find it difficult to be straightforward about this. Instead, they just override the patient's wishes.

On other occasions, a kind of manipulation goes on. The practitioner tricks the client into having something done, for example in order to fulfil a quota for audit or income purposes, while making it seem as if they are doing the client an unsolicited favour. It is preferable to strategise openly by saying "I'm sorry to suggest this at an inappropriate moment, but part of my job is to get these things done."

Not following feedback

Practitioner: When did the problem start?
Client: As soon as I came back from my holiday.
Practitioner: When exactly was that?

This conversation represents a missed opportunity. By sticking rigidly to the bald facts of chronology, the interviewer has missed something that might be important. What is the significance of the holiday in the patient's story? Could something have happened on the holiday that gave rise to "the problem," or was it the effects of coming back that may have been associated with it? Are there lessons to be learned from what has happened after previous holidays, or previous returns home? Of course, there might not be, but the interviewer will never know without asking questions such as "Was there any reason it happened exactly at that time?"

Not tracking language

Practitioner: Did what you try make a difference?
Client: Yes, to an extent.
Practitioner: Good, so can you carry on?

In some ways, this is a subtler version of not following feedback. What the interviewer is missing here is the precise nuances of language. The practitioner has chosen to accept the part of the client's utterance that is positive, but ignored a more ambiguous phrase ("to an extent"). If unpacked, this phrase might turn out to disguise considerable reservations about what has happened. What is the gap between what was desired and what actually happened? Would inquiry into this gap reveal that the positive tone arises from diffidence, respect, or fear rather than frankness? Interestingly, one notices these nuances far more as an observer than a participant in an interview. Being observed by one's peers in training exercises also appears to hone the ability to be attentive to language, and to reflect on an appropriate response such as "So how did it make a difference . . . And did it fall short in any way?"

Being wedded to your hypothesis

Practitioner: Does any particular type of event trigger your panic attack?
Client: I don't think so. No.
Practitioner: Try to remember. It's quite common for these attacks to have a pattern.

Professionals often have quite strong beliefs about the nature and origins of particular problems. They are often so concerned to establish that their assumptions or hypotheses are the correct ones that they may find it quite difficult to notice when a patient is uninterested, puzzled or even affronted by them. Naturally, there are some instances where it is appropriate to probe beyond an initial rejection of a hypothesis. Indeed, sometimes clients later agree with a hypothesis they strongly rejected at first. On the other hand, pushing a hypothesis too hard can alienate the other person. It is usually better to let a previous assumption go as soon as it appears to have no use for the person sitting in front of you at that moment, and offer a more open-minded approach: "Do you have any ideas yourself about what triggers them?"

Psychologising

Practitioner:	Do you think your problems are made worse at all by stress?
Client:	I really don't think so.
Practitioner:	But I'm aware you do find your job very stressful at the moment.

One of the commonest forms of being wedded to a hypothesis is psychologising. This is probably a manifestation of the widespread belief among health and social care professionals that everything must have "an underlying cause," and that psychological underlying causes are more important and profound than anything else. This may in some cases be true, but what is often problematical is the practitioner's implicit claim to know that this is the case even in the face of the client's clear assertion that it is not. Such a claim privileges the professional's assumptions over the client's language, and can amount to an abuse of power, compared with more neutral inquires such as "What other factors in your life might be relevant?"

Unsolicited interpretations

Practitioner:	I really lost my rag with my boss again last week, and I am in pretty deep water as a result.
Interviewer:	Does this hark back to anything in your family background?

Psychological theories have made their way into health and social care to such an extent they are sometimes used in fairly "wild" ways. A common habit, as here, is to assume that anything that elicits strong feeling must refer back to someone else from the past, probably a parent. Incidentally, professionals also tend to do this to each other when consulting on cases, for example suggesting that a particular patient has been upset because of triggering unpleasant personal memories. Clearly, there are instances where this may be the case. However, rather than jumping on a potentially raw nerve with both feet, it is usually more appropriate to ask patients to propose their own hypotheses concerning the causes of problems, such as "Can you tell me anything about why this keeps happening?"

Dwelling on emotions, especially negative ones

Practitioner: How do you feel about having had a stroke?
Client: Bloody awful at the time, but I'm feeling a lot better now that my strength has come back.
Practitioner: But you must have felt very frightened and angry at first.

Both professional and popular culture in the past century have encouraged the expression of strong negative emotion, often on the assumption that it will lead in almost any circumstances to catharsis and relief. Our own observation is that this is very rarely the case, unless it is done with great skill and in protected therapeutic settings. Far more often, we see a rather clumsy attempt to summon or recreate painful feelings in a consulting context where issues of timing, resources or the other tasks that need to be addressed mean that this is inappropriate. The problem with such attempts is that they allow the other person no choice as to whether they want to explore feelings of this kind. While there may be some occasions when they do wish to express or discharge strong emotion, there is always the danger that they may feel obliged to respond in this way against their will. One way of avoiding this is to pose the choice neutrally, with a question such as "Do you want to talk a bit more about how it felt then, or would you prefer to say where you are now?"

We also counsel against the repeated use of reframing, with phrases such as "It sounds to me as if . . . " Although many practitioners use this technique as a routine, we have often seen clients react to this as if the practitioner is "taking over" the story, or closing it down by replacing the original words with others that do not fit as well. Similarly, many practitioners seem to fall back on the question "How did you feel about that?" when they cannot think of anything else to say. In practice, the question often seems to halt the progress of any narrative by amplifying the negative feelings connected with the problem rather than seeking a way forward.

One metaphor that many find useful in this regard is to see narrative practice as less like peeling an onion and more like weaving a tapestry. Another helpful idea is to regard the conversation not as a vertical exercise (such as digging a hole), but more of a horizontal one (such as travelling across a landscape.) In keeping with this, we promote more neutral forms of questioning such as "What impact is this having on you now?"

Giving advice disguised as questioning

Practitioner: Had you thought of telling your mother you can't visit so often?
Client: No, not really, I don't think she could cope.
Practitioner: But would you consider trying it anyway?

Most practitioners nowadays know that they rarely have the right simply to tell others what to do. On the other hand, the temptation to give advice is irresistible, and it is fairly easy to package advice in the form of questions that pose as neutral but are really not. Once again, there may often be a place for exploring how different options could be tried out, but this may best be done in neutral forms of words that implicitly give the patient as much permission to reject as to accept the advice. For example, in the case above, it would be possible to enquire:

- "What effect do you think it would have if you told your mother you were going in less?"
- "How would she show that she wasn't really coping with the prospect of reduced visits?"

Compulsive explaining

Client: I've never really understood why I need oxygen at home.
Practitioner: Well, let me explain again what your hospital report says . . .

Many professionals are thoroughly committed to an educational approach in their everyday work. They may see explanations as intrinsically empowering, and therefore an essential part of every encounter with a patient. However, explanations can be problematical, as this example shows. They may pre-empt any attempt to elicit someone's own understanding first. For example, does the person here really have no rudimentary idea that might be worth exploring first? If an explanation has been given previously, what led to the persisting state of bewilderment? Often, interviewers give accounts of conditions and treatments in a way that is well-meaning, but simply does not relate to the recipients' levels of understanding, their capacity to take in information, or their anxiety. The only way practitioners can orient themselves to ask the right questions is by first checking out where patients or clients are to start with: "Can you just run through what you understand about your condition, and I can try to fill in any gaps . . . "

The wish to change people

Client: I really need help with my knees.
Practitioner: Well, I have mentioned before about the importance of losing weight.

There is universal acceptance that professionals have an important role in prevention and risk reduction. At the same time, they are often ill-equipped to manage conversations with those who cannot change or do not want to. The example here shows a practitioner who is unable to respond to the fact that previous advice about change has not been effective. As a result, there is no acknowledgement of the statement that something is "needed," except with an implied reproach. What is missing is a frank negotiation about what is possible and why, and what is impossible and why: "At some point, I'd like to talk about your weight again. Is this a good moment or do you want to focus on other things first?"

Suggested exercises

1 After any conversation, try to recall any question or statement that seemed to impede the dialogue, and try to identify how this prevented the kind of dialogue you wished for.
2 When you are not too busy, observe yourself in a series of conversations. Which of your conversational habits slow down others' stories, and which of them help the stories flow more freely?

CHAPTER FIVE

Helping narratives to develop

Key ideas in this chapter

- There are some straightforward ways of encouraging the development of clients' narratives.
- It is possible to adopt conversational techniques that invite more helpful and coherent narratives while still carrying out the appropriate professional task.
- Narrative-based practice can be adapted for challenging encounters, including those where clients do not speak English, or when there are disagreements.

Introduction

This chapter offers some specific guidance about actively helping clients to develop new accounts of their experiences and difficulties. It also looks at ways of integrating a wide range of familiar activities in health and social care into narrative-based practice. These suggestions are not meant as inflexible guidelines. Practitioners who try out narrative ideas commonly discover how to use certain patterns of behaviour and speech that some of their colleagues find helpful in their turn, while others may not. Using these techniques can also feel a little unnatural at first. However, we find that they soon become integrated into practitioners' natural ways of communicating, so that clients may notice nothing unusual about them apart from the fact that they encourage more open responses. The ideas presented here are a compendium of hints and tips that we have built up collaboratively over time, in response to questions that professionals bring about narrative-based practice. These are illustrated with case examples that learners and practitioners have described, suitably anonymised.

How should I prepare for any meeting or consultation?

Many narrative practitioners have adopted the habit of reading the referral letter, previous notes or computer record before any appointment, in order to familiarise themselves with "the story so far." This usually gives rise to some spontaneous hypotheses and questions. It can be especially useful to try to give hypotheses a definite shape rather than a vague one: for example, what are the possible or likely developments since the referral or last appointment took place, and what might be useful questions to pursue to explore these? Although new learners inevitably fear this can be time-consuming, in practice they often find it makes the use of time in the conversation itself more efficient. The quality of the reflective space that any professional manages to set aside in advance of an encounter, however brief, may determine the possibilities for new narratives to develop. Apart from anything else, it means that patients or clients are far more likely to feel known and understood from the beginning of an encounter, and provides the conditions for attentiveness and eye contact from the start.

Fetching a person or family from the waiting area gives opportunities for further possibilities to come to mind, perhaps based on body language or on the particular combination of family members who have turned up for a meeting. Home visits offer even more opportunities for picking up cues with all of the senses and may then inform the conversations that take place there.

A practitioner reported:

In the past, I never looked at the notes or the computer before calling someone through. I thought there just wasn't the time. However, I've now started doing it. Last week, I saw a woman who lost her husband a year ago, and when I looked at her notes I realised it was the first anniversary of his death – the exact day. She was really touched that I was aware of this. It was extraordinary that I had noticed, and it transformed the meeting.

How should I open a conversation?

In many pre-planned encounters, such as social care assessments or health care reviews, it helps to establish clarity about the exact purpose of the conversation at the outset, for example with a question such as "Can I just check why you think we're meeting up today?" Surprisingly often, service users may have a quite different understanding of the purpose of the encounter from the one that the professional assumed was obvious.

In more open-ended appointments, a conventional question such as "How can I help you?" or "What has brought you here today?" is fine from a narrative point of view, although some practitioners prefer to say nothing, and find that an expectant facial expression alone will bring forth the client's first statement. We counsel against the use of formulations such as "What's the problem?" since this already closes down some possibilities (for example, there may not be a problem, or there may be several).

What about taking notes or entering them in the computer?

In order to signal an emphasis on oral narrative, it seems helpful to keep note-taking during any conversation to a minimum. As well as detracting from eye contact or sitting face-to-face, taking notes lessens the amount of attentiveness available for the other person, and the opportunity for reflection on the part of the practitioner. Clearly, there are situations when practitioners do need to jot some things down, but it is perfectly possible to do this as rough notes and transfer the details to the main written record or computer screen afterwards. To lessen distraction, it even helps to have the computer screen switched off (or showing a neutral screen saver) during the consultation.

Some learners say they cannot imagine running on time unless they write records at the same time as consulting. However, most practitioners find that uninterrupted attention makes things move along more quickly, so that there is enough time left over for making records afterwards – or for quickly running through whatever then has to be done to meet bureaucratic demands. In addition, writing the notes afterwards may make it possible to construct a more concise and focused account of what has passed. It can also be useful to include some brief information about the conversational process itself in the notes, particularly if this may point towards useful questions that can be raised at the next encounter with the patient.

How can I think of lots of good questions to help narratives develop?

This is a very common question from people learning a narrative-based approach. It is tempting to offer a vast and comprehensive checklist in response but, as explained in the previous chapter, this would be counterproductive. It could lead to highly stylised interviews, undertaken by rote instead of through following feedback. Nevertheless, a few principles appear to help people develop good questioning and a facility in crafting new ones:

- Pick up words or phrases that the patient has just said, using these as a starting point for further inquiry.
- Focus on developing a general sense of process and circularity in the interview, rather than worrying about technical prowess.
- If a question doesn't yield useful information, don't repeat it. Ask a different one, or just wait and see what happens.
- Keep questions short. Don't add long explanations to each question. Ask one at a time, not a whole catalogue.
- Monitor your own questioning and see how you can make them fit better with the other person's narrative flow.
- Pay attention to how colleagues (and even radio or TV interviewers) ask different kinds of questions, and the effect this has on opening the narrative up or closing it down.
- If the patient answers a question you didn't ask, go with the flow!
- Over time, build up your own collection of effective questions – by trial and error, by observing others at work, and by reading. Consider making a record of these.

One of the most effective ways of helping narratives forward is to ask questions that draw attention to the underlying values or beliefs that appear to be guiding people's behaviour. An example of this might be "You say your husband feels your disability is less than you think. What might give him a different view?" Although elaborate questions such as this can seem unwieldy at first, they can prompt powerful results if well thought-out and if you have judged the timing appropriately.

A practitioner explained:

I regularly see a young man who seems depressed and also rather isolated. He often tells me about how people have let him down: family, friends, social workers, the Citizens Advice Bureau, and so on. Last week, he came in with another catalogue of disappointments. It occurred to me to ask him if he could think of any occasions recently when someone actually provided something he had asked for, and also whether he'd ever been able to influence anyone to do this. The question made him think. He couldn't recall anything then and there, but said he'd chew over it before the next time he sees me.

How can you do things such as completing questionnaires, or carrying out a physical examination, while maintaining a narrative stance?

Technical tasks can disrupt the narrative flow of an encounter. However, disruption can be lessened by seeking permission, and offering an explanation:

- "I need to go through some questions to see if you might be entitled to extra benefits. Is this a good moment to do this?"
- "Is it all right if I listen to your chest at this point?"

Although such questions can seem rather precious at first, they are useful because they set a context for what the practitioner is doing. This enhances the sense of collaboration. A physical examination can also allow time for silent reflection, and almost every doctor or nurse will confess to using a stethoscope to buy time in order to reflect on the conversation so far or form hypotheses and questions for the next stage.

What about prescribing?

Many health professionals write prescriptions as part of a strategy for bringing the patient's story to a close. There are obviously better ways of integrating a prescription into the narrative. From a narrative point of view, offering a prescription is just a suggestion for taking the conversation in one particular direction, and therefore open to further discussion. There are many occasions when it makes sense to declare a strong opinion either way about the need for medication or aids, and practitioners can still make this clear without foreclosing the narrative. However, the prescription needs to end up fitting the story, rather than the other way round. From a narrative perspective, there is nothing intrinsically right or wrong about prescribing antibiotics for conditions where this might be considered debatable. What matters is whether or not the clinician has created a context for discussing this.

A practitioner explained:

In the past, I used to get into serious tussles with parents about antibiotics for kids with colds. What I tend to do now is say "Look, the child specialists tell us not to give antibiotics for colds, but a lot of parents feel helpless if they don't have something to give." I explained this to a mother last week and she said "That's the real problem. But if I know it isn't going to help, I'd rather not give it."

How can a label or diagnosis fit in with the narrative?

From a narrative point of view, a label or diagnosis of a problem is a form of story, albeit a highly respectable one that may command general agreement among professionals. Being given a name for a problem may be useful to someone and have a great deal of meaning for them (because, for example, they already know someone else who has a condition with that name). It may also help because it places them within a community of others with the same condition, and gives them a common language to use with the professionals they encounter.

The most important aspect of a diagnosis or any form of categorisation is that it has an inescapable effect on the narrative itself. The act of naming alters what is named, and how it is experienced (von Schlippe, 2001). Sometimes, giving a name to a condition makes it seem more manageable (e.g. "Now I know my son has a learning disability, I can get the right kind of help"). At other times, it can make the condition seem more intractable (e.g. "Well if he's autistic, he's stuck with it for life"). For a diagnosis to be helpful, the positive effects on the narrative must outweigh the negative. It also needs to be the starting point for the next episode of the story rather than a form of foreclosure. As many others have pointed out, there also needs to be a distinction between the condition and the whole person: very few patients appreciate being described, for example, as "diabetics" or "epileptics."

There are risks to giving labels too. Diagnoses and formulations can be so familiar to professionals that it is easy to lose sight of how they can have different meanings – or none at all – to the individuals who are given them. They can also close down any further discussion of someone's unique experience of that condition, or the beliefs and ideas that accompany that experience. For that reason, it can be useful to have a repertoire of questions that can accompany any diagnosis that is proffered. These include questions such as:

- "What would be the benefits and disadvantages of using the word 'disabled' about yourself?"
- "What do you understand by 'Alzheimer's,' and what would you like me to explain about it?"
- "When you were told you were 'partially sighted,' what difference did that make? How?"

- "Has anyone else called this 'asthma'? How helpful was it?"
- "How well does the word 'depression' fit your experience?"

In many circumstances, especially with "grey area" conditions, it can be more helpful to offer what has been called a "narrative diagnosis," in effect a short story that better reflects the practitioner's uncertainty than any attempt to categorise something that may not be categorisable. For example, the following account might be given to patients as an alternative to saying they have "irritable bowel syndrome" (Launer, 2012):

> I can't find anything physically wrong with you and the tests haven't shown anything. Your symptoms are pretty common and don't to point to anything major. Some doctors like to call this kind of thing "irritable bowel syndrome." It's fine for you to choose whether you like the term or not. Either way, there are several different kinds of medication that might help, and there are dietary changes that may make a difference too.

Is it possible to give advice within narrative-based practice?

No one could possibly work in health and social care without giving advice and information a great deal of the time. From the point of view of narrative, the crucial issue is whether this is given in response to how the story is already evolving, or whether it hijacks the conversation. Whenever possible, it is helpful to reframe every piece of advice as a suggestion, and therefore as part of a dialogue rather than a monologue. One way that this can be done is by packaging advice within a question such as "What do you think would happen if you tried . . . ?" or "Something that people often seem to find useful in this situation is . . . Do you think that might work in your case?" However, this technique will fail unless the practitioner is committed to paying attention to the answer – even if it is an entirely negative one – and picking up the narrative thread from that point. It can also be disingenuous, for example if you know that someone has no option except to follow the recommendation set by a court or other external authority.

There are other occasions when practitioners have to give very strong advice for purely ethical reasons. For example, a hospital doctor who has just diagnosed peritonitis does not want to sound as if the recommendation for an immediate operation is tentative, or requires a long and reflective discussion. Yet even on these relatively unusual occasions, it is still possible to put very assertive advice in dialogical form: "I am going to have to tell you something you may find a bit alarming . . . but I'll make sure you have enough time to respond and ask any questions you want."

How can I bring evidence into the narrative?

Evidence-based practice has become one of the dominant ideas in recent years. However, it is an idea – one might say a kind of narrative in its own right – that often does not have an easy correspondence with the stories that are brought into the consulting room. The following two case examples are designed to show how tensions between evidence and narrative can express themselves. Each is followed by a commentary pointing towards ways that these tensions might be lessened.

Case example: exhausted parents

Mr and Mrs J are a couple whose son Jake, age 2, has severe eczema. Jake's parents say they are frantic at their inability to stop Jake scratching, and also because of sleep deprivation. The practitioner knows they should be giving Jake daily baths, and applying copious amounts of moisturisers – something that all the evidence shows will improve his skin condition. When she asks about this, however, their response is one of despondency. They cannot imagine fitting the regime of meticulous skincare into their lives, especially as they also have a 4-year-old and a new baby.

Commentary

The tension here between narrative and evidence may arise because the parents' narrative is not just about Jake's eczema, but about their own helplessness and exhaustion. The way to reach a convergence of stories might be for the practitioner to set aside her own chosen narrative of Jake's skincare and to concentrate instead on their unmanageable feelings. Interpolating limited amounts of evidence-based information into a dialogue about his condition is likely to be far more effective than a mini-seminar on skincare guidelines.

Case example: untreated blood pressure

Mrs M is a 45-year-old woman with raised blood pressure and other risk factors, including being obese. Her mother died of a stroke at the age of 50. The practitioner has entered all her risk factors onto his surgery computer, and this gives her nearly a 30 per cent risk of a heart attack or stroke in the next 10 years.

Mrs M says that she is not surprised as she has a lot of stress in her job as a hospital orderly. However, she believes the problem cannot be as serious as her mother's because she does not suffer from headaches in the way her mother always did. She says she will try to lose weight just by cutting out bread and potatoes, but she is not keen to take drugs because she is sure they will make her feel nauseated just as any medication always does.

Commentary

It is conventional to look at the practitioner's version in a case such as this as the true reality of the situation, and to dismiss the patient's account as ignorant, confused, or the result of denial. However, it may be more useful to look at these two versions of reality as parallel narratives. The doctor has one story inside his head that has been influenced by his own past encounters and life experiences in the same way as Mrs M. If he tries to persuade her to adopt this in its entirety, he may be no more likely to succeed than if she tried to convert him to hers. If he wins a technical success and she takes the drugs, she may do so with a sense of enduring disempowerment or resentment.

By thinking of this encounter as a mismatch of narratives, the practitioner may open up the possibility of a new account that both parties can subscribe to. Does Mrs M know, for example, of anyone who has taken medication for blood pressure without ill effects? Conversely, can the practitioner remember anyone such as Mrs M who did lose weight and manage without medication?

How can I fit in health and safety promotion?

Given the contemporary emphasis on risk reduction and the long-term management of conditions, it would be unprofessional to distract practitioners from attending to these. The crucial issue is about doing this transparently. While professionals may feel they should be as persuasive as possible, the clients they deal with may experience this as paternalistic and authoritarian, unless they are given information about the context in which advice is being offered. If, for instance, a health check needs to be done because the clinic protocol says it should, or because there are financial rewards or penalties attached, it may help to declare this context. Clients can then decide how to respond to this from their own personal perspective.

A nurse said:

> I hate all the things I have to do to patients these days. I feel it stops me being a proper nurse and turns me into a kind of civil servant. I was so exasperated last week that I said this to a patient. I was surprised by her reaction. She said she always appreciated it when I checked her blood pressure, or checked her records for smears and so on – even when she hadn't asked me to. For her, it was a sign I was a really good nurse because I thought about her needs, even ones she didn't know about. I had felt rather ashamed of blurting out my feelings, but learned something important as a result.

How can I use a narrative approach with people who don't speak English?

Most professionals in health and social care have a considerable caseload of individuals and families who do not speak English, and who attend either with relatives who interpret for them, or with paid interpreters, link workers or advocates. In some ways, this can be seen as an obstacle or complicating factor in encounters. In another way, it is also possible to see it as a unique opportunity for applying a narrative approach. For example, the time taken to translate each utterance may allow the practitioner additional time for reflection, and for preparing the next stage of the conversation.

Family members or even interpreters may have their own ideas to contribute, and if this is handled ethically, it can enrich the conversation rather than impoverishing it. If interpreters are from the client's own country, for example, they may be able to provide important contextual information about cultural traditions and expectations. Clients from many ethnic backgrounds may expect that other family members or friends present in the room will in any case be involved in decision-making, and may be unfamiliar with the dyadic exchanges that are more common in their adopted country. Clearly, these matters need to be handled with appropriate sensitivity and with respect to the client's own autonomy, so that others do not take over the encounter without consent, but more often than not clients may appreciate such multidimensional exchanges.

How can I manage people who bring multiple problems?

This can be seen as a shared problem for practitioner and client. Most patients and clients are aware that a professional's time is limited, and that the work needs to be focused. The key for managing this well seems to be to strategise the encounter jointly with the patient, and to strategise early. This might involve, for example, checking out at the very beginning of the conversation whether more than one problem has to be addressed, and to share the preliminary work of time management with the patient:

- "Are these all part of the same problem, or do we need to go about them one by one?"
- "Supposing we only have time today to deal with one of these, which is the most pressing?"

Time and its limitations generally go unmentioned in professional encounters, but there is absolutely no reason why this should be so, and there are many reasons to challenge this convention:

- "We're running out of time shortly. Is there anything important we haven't covered or might need to revisit another time?"

The next example shows an unusually imaginative use of questioning that could possibly never be reproduced, but turned out to fit the moment exactly.
A practitioner told us:

A man came in and said "I've got four problems." I asked him "Is there a fifth?" I did this intuitively, without even thinking. I've never done this before and I'm not sure I'd ever do it again, but something in his face led me to ask it. He obviously understood what had happened because he said yes and he told me about it. It was the most important problem, and we spent the whole consultation talking about it. He seemed to forget the other problems. I'm not sure what made me take the risk and ask him something so bold. It may have been his body language, or just intuition.

How can I deal with people who bring inappropriate problems?

Most professionals encounter clients who have brought problems that seem more appropriate for other professionals or other agencies. They may have attended mainly because a service is accessible and free, or because their understanding of complex institutional structures and professional boundaries is limited. Perhaps what they really need is a lawyer, a benefits advisor, a housing officer, or their MP. Often, service users may subscribe to a view of professionals being part of the social establishment, and therefore possessing a great deal of influence and power, whereas practitioners themselves are more likely to have a narrative about their own work that emphasises lack of resources, poor or limited access to other agencies, and powerlessness outside a fairly narrow set of professional connections. Somehow, the gap between the two narratives needs to be bridged in a way that avoids confrontation.

The following strategy seems to be realistic and respectful in this situation:

- Inquiry into the person's story of need and helplessness without prematurely foreclosing it.
- Responding with information concerning what other agencies can and should offer, rather than what your own agency cannot. For many practitioners, this sometimes involves advising others how to negotiate with an inflexible bureaucracy or an under-resourced agency, in order to ensure that their needs and rights are met.
- Further questioning about the person's response to the advice.

A practitioner said:

> A woman came to see me, desperate to get her daughter into the local grammar school – rather than the one nearest her that has a terrible reputation. She wanted me to write a report saying her child had all sorts of special educational needs, but there really wasn't anything in her notes to justify this. I had seen the daughter previously, but it was about a behaviour problem and this had settled. In the end, I managed to have a conversation with her that wasn't really about her daughter at all, but about racial discrimination and about how she felt she'd never had a chance herself educationally. I couldn't write a report, but I hope she felt able to take on the system better and work out a way of getting her girl into the school she wants.

How can I manage disagreement or hostility?

Few practitioners in health and social care can avoid encounters where they face disagreement and hostility. Professionals may carry a responsibility to make judgements about such matters as child protection or entitlement to services and benefits. These judgements will sometimes be at variance with what service users expect or regard as fair. From a narrative point of view, there are two particularly unhelpful strategies when such disagreements arise. The first is to try to foreclose any discussion arbitrarily without allowing the other person to express their view – a response that is only likely to heighten tension and provoke more anger. The other risk is to try to seek an amicable resolution by prolonging the conversation way beyond the point where there is any possibility of resolution.

While there are no hard and fast rules for making such encounters more comfortable, a narrative-based approach would generally follow these principles:

- Explaining dispassionately that your judgement is based on clear external guidance about how to make such decisions.
- Allowing sufficient time for the other person to express the reasons for their disagreement, and to accept their narrative as legitimate from their own point of view, even if it cannot override the decision.
- Explaining what recourse is open to them if they want to challenge your judgement.

As with the earlier examples of situations where there is a mismatch of narratives between the practitioner and the service user, it is worth bearing in mind that neither narrative may be right or wrong in absolute terms, but simply that there are circumstances where the practitioner has been assigned the power to apply established rules and override the other person's judgement, and has no choice but to do so.

An optometrist explained:

A man of around 70 came for a routine eye check and it was clear at once that his vision was far below an acceptable level for driving, and glasses or surgery could never correct this. I told him, and I don't think I have ever seen anyone so angry in my life. He said he adamantly refused to inform the driving authorities, so I advised him I would have to do so instead. He shouted at me for about 10 minutes about how I had ruined his life as he depended on driving in order to visit his children in another city and his cottage in the country. I allowed him as much time as I could to express how upset he was about this. In the end, we managed to agree on two things: first, that he could bring his son the next week for a further discussion, and also that I would refer him to the hospital for a second opinion, even though I knew this would only lead to the same outcome. Obviously, I could not alter my decision about informing the licensing authority as he was a danger to other road users.

How can I do all of this and still run to time?

Most people who are trying out narrative techniques for the first time report that they are held up in their consultations. This is perhaps inevitable as part of the learning process, and learners need to make allowances for it. On the positive side, once learners have acquired proficiency, they usually report that they are much more adept at keeping within time boundaries than they ever were previously. One reason may be that they become more confident about making time limitations explicit, and about sharing decisions about time management.

Many practitioners who have adopted a narrative-based approach realise how ridiculous it is to try to cram an almost limitless agenda of six or seven problems, screening, advice and empathic counselling all into a few minutes. They then discover how to share an account of their constraints with clients, in a descriptive rather than confrontational manner, and to collaborate in setting priorities, or by doing things in stages, or thinking about other resources elsewhere. Also, they may no longer strive to achieve the impossible, because they have a more realistic sense of the contexts that govern and constrain their work.

How should I end a narrative-based conversation?

If all goes well in a conversation, an appropriate ending will become apparent to the participants rather than having to be imposed arbitrarily. However, in reality, there is often not enough time to address all of someone's needs. There are ways of making this clear. It is perfectly acceptable to say "I'm afraid we do need to finish for today." With practice, it is easily possible to make such statements in an entirely friendly and non-confrontational way, although it is surprising how nervous and guilt-ridden practitioners can be about doing so for the first time. An invitation to choose the interval of time before the next encounter can help to bring about a negotiated ending. In an effective narrative-based conversation, clients will quite often bring an encounter to a close spontaneously themselves with a comment such as "I didn't really know what I thought until I heard myself say it," "I suppose I knew all along what I needed to do," or even "I never really thought it was a big problem in the first place." Although the professional may feel that he or she has played an important part in facilitating this narrative reconstruction, it rarely helps to point this out. Modesty, and satisfaction at rendering one's techniques invisible, are probably more appropriate.

Suggested exercises

1 Review an encounter and consider how "conventional" activity such as a diagnosis, formulation or advice were incorporated into the narrative. Were there other ways this might have been done? What would the possible effects have been?

2 Consider the rules or habits you adopt as your "conversational etiquette" (e.g. the way you summon clients, the position you sit in, how you take notes, etc.). How far do these impede or facilitate narrative development? How might you change them? Could you make a video recording of yourself at work and review this?

References

Launer, J. (2012) Narrative diagnosis. *Postgraduate Medical Journal*, 88(1036), 115–116.

von Schlippe, A. (2001) Talking about asthma: the semantic environments of physical disease. *Families, Systems and Health*, 19, 251–262.

CHAPTER SIX

Families

Key ideas in this chapter

- For most patients and clients, families play a central part in how they understand and experience their problems. Inquiry into the family dimension of their lives is often an essential part of a narrative approach.
- There are specific ways of bringing the family into people's narratives, including circular questions and the use of genograms (family trees).
- Taking genograms is not a formidable exercise. It can be short, simple and highly effective. Practitioners can easily adopt it as a routine narrative tool.
- Health and social care offer enormous scope for working with families, whether the problem is an individual one or a shared family one. Such work can be brief and integrated with everyday care.

Introduction

Family stories are nearly always present in the room, even if only one person is there with you physically. Family members are present in the life stories that people carry inside their heads. They are also there in remembered or imagined conversations. Many narratives brought to professionals will have been rehearsed in advance with someone in the family. Most conversations with practitioners will in turn become the material of a further story, told to the family at home afterwards. Our stories, and our identities themselves, are quintessentially family ones. This chapter is about the family dimension of people's narratives. It looks at how to apply narrative-based practice when there is only one client in the room and the conversation takes a family perspective, but also addresses encounters with two or more family members at the same time. The anonymised case examples are taken from practitioners who have applied a narrative-based approach in their everyday work, using a family perspective.

Exploring personal identity through family history

It is sometimes only possible to make sense of an individual's problem by inquiring into the family conversations that have previously taken place. Some of the most revealing questions in the narrative practitioner's repertoire include the following:

- "Who at home is most worried about your problem?"
- "Was it your decision to come today or did someone else suggest it?"
- "Have you talked about this problem to anyone in your family? What did they make of it?"

Equally, it is sometimes only possible to develop or consolidate a new story by finding out who else needs to be involved in the process:

- "What would help to reassure your daughter that this wasn't a serious illness?"
- "How do you think you might explain what is going on to family and friends?"
- "Who is going to need the most convincing that you're looking after yourself properly?"

There are, however, many conversations when it helps to go beyond such questions and to explore a fuller picture of clients' family backgrounds. Although some health and social care practitioners feel inhibited about making a family inquiry a routine part of their professional encounters, this is rarely experienced as an intrusion. Few of us define ourselves by our medical or social histories. We generally see ourselves more as the children of our parents, or the parents of our children, or as siblings or spouses, partners, or members of a more extended family. Moreover, individual adversity often has a profound impact on the family. A family inquiry can be introduced with a question as simple as "Can I ask a bit about your family background?" or "Who's at home these days?" If the verbal or non-verbal response indicates that such inquiries are unwelcome, they can easily be dropped. To make it entirely clear that the motive is not one of looking for someone to blame for a problem, it may be useful to add "I find it helps me to understand people more if I know who's around in their lives."

Asking questions about the family is often the best way of moving from the professional's perspective of the story to the client's. However, it is particularly powerful in developing a new story when other, more conventional methods are proving unproductive. Family inquiry is therefore particularly useful with depression, somatisation, behavioural problems, dependency on drugs or alcohol, relationship difficulties, or previous failed interventions (Asen et al., 2003). It can also help when either client or professional feel stuck.

The following case shows how well, and how economically, such an approach can sometimes work.

Case example: Hassan P

A practitioner said:

> I was struggling to make a connection with a young Kurdish man, Hassan. He was an asylum seeker and I was trying to help him claim some benefits. He gave one-word answers to all my questions, even though his English seemed quite good. So I decided to stop filling in the computer template for a couple of minutes and asked him about his family instead. He told me that he had left his parents and five siblings behind in Iraq. I asked "Are they all safe?" He suddenly became highly animated. I felt it transformed the quality of the consultation.

Genograms: the basic tool for creating family narratives

Most family therapists take genograms (family trees) as a routine. Many practitioners in health and social care are reluctant to do so. The main worry seems to be that they cannot possibly record all the details of a family in the time available so should not even start it. However, if the basic task of taking a genogram is seen as a way of eliciting more of someone's story, only a very few questions may be needed to accomplish this effectively. The formal phrase "taking a genogram" should not deter anyone from jotting down an improvised diagram in a few seconds on a piece of scrap paper, which can amount to exactly the same thing. Figure 6.1 shows the basic symbols for writing down a genogram. For enthusiasts, computer software is available for including genograms in electronic records.

Case example: Harold B

A practitioner explained:

> A man of 78, Harold B, was telling me about unaccountable feelings of sadness and failure. These had appeared fairly suddenly the previous month. Nothing in his circumstances seemed to account for this. Everything in his family and life seemed to be going so well. His oldest grandchild had just reached the age of 10. I asked him a few questions

about his family. He told me that his own grandfather had died just after his tenth birthday – the same age his grandson had just reached! He was stunned when he made the connection. He burst out with all kinds of ideas. He realised how scared he was of dying himself now. It was a quite dramatic consultation.

Trying out a new story

In one way, a genogram just establishes the bare bones of someone's life story. However, from a narrative point of view, it is the creative act itself – the live

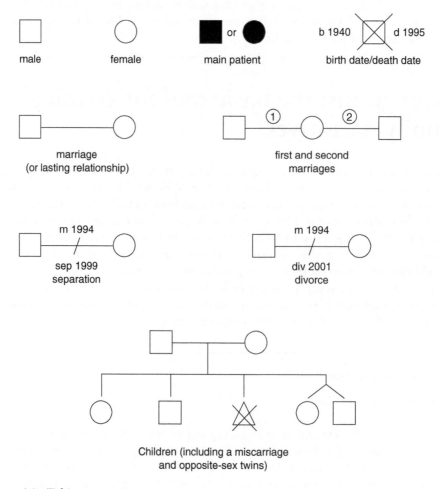

Children (including a miscarriage
and opposite-sex twins)

Figure 6.1 Taking a genogram

construction of a genogram between practitioner and service user – that is crucial. It not only creates intimacy, but brings about new understanding and indeed new stories about how the past came to influence and determine the present. Giving a coherent account of the past, and how it came to influence current difficulties, can help others to identify what needs to be changed so that they can create a different story for themselves.

Case example: Karen N

A practitioner told us:

> I have been seeing a woman called Karen N regularly while she has been going through a series of treatments for breast cancer. She has had a mastectomy, radiotherapy and chemotherapy. She keeps telling me about how she cannot stop being a "coper." She is always looking after everyone else, including her husband and two teenagers, and a disabled daughter. She finds it impossible to take as much rest as she needs, even though her family seem fairly willing to help. I recently asked her a few questions about her family of origin. She was the eldest of five children. Her father was confined to bed for all of her teenage years because of spinal tuberculosis. She was effectively brought up as her mother's "right hand." She said it was hard to let go of control. We talked about this and drew up a genogram together. She realised that her present family set-up is far more supportive than the one she was brought up with. She is going to try to let others do more for her.

Taking genograms as a routine

Many practitioners will think nothing of taking down elaborate past medical or social histories or health screening information for every new person they see. Yet many probably find the idea of taking genograms systematically rather intimidating. This need not be the case. It probably takes much less time to elicit a basic family story than it does to fill in the average computer template for a newly registered patient or client. It may be far more effective in terms of the quantity and quality of information gathered.

Taking genograms leads to a more rounded understanding of the stories of many patients, especially those who are seen mainly in terms of their diseases or other superficial characteristics. It also makes it possible to see important connections between individuals who seemed unconnected – for example, married sisters with different surnames, or fathers and their married daughters – and to learn of significant members of the household. It often produces important stories unexpectedly, especially when practitioners have become so familiarised with people that they have developed unvarying stories about them. Perhaps because of this, routine taking of genograms seems to produce a strongly positive effect on one's perception of others. It can also sometimes reveal a family history of risk factors when this has been missed by other routine screening systems.

Systematic taking of genograms also helps to focus attention more on families with particularly troubling stories to tell. These include:

- early or repeated separations and disruptions in childhood;
- the concurrence of two or more significant new problems in the same household in a short space of time;
- a family history of widespread major psychiatric disorder;
- childlessness and consequent isolation in the elderly, particularly useful in cases where the professional has erroneously assumed that there was another generation of potential family carers;
- existence of a previous marriage or partnership, and sometimes also of resulting children from whom the person might now be estranged;
- early parental death;
- a history of immigration or emigration within the family;
- a history of persecution and fleeing, with consequent separation from spouses, parents or children; and
- unconventional households (for example, elderly single brothers living together).

However, there can also be drawbacks to taking genograms in an organised way. Like stamp collecting or trainspotting, there is a risk that it can turn into an obsession that distracts practitioners from the primary purpose of enlarging their understanding. It requires discipline to recall that the point of taking genograms in a professional context is for their power to create new stories, not for the amassing of data in itself, as the following cautionary example shows.

Case example: Irene M

A learner wrote:

> I saw an adolescent girl, Irene M, whose weight loss strongly suggested the early presentation of an eating disorder. I started a genogram with her. She became extremely enthusiastic about the idea and went home to construct an enormous six-generation genogram on a sheet of unused wallpaper. She returned with her mother a fortnight later, and proudly showed me the genogram. We had a long discussion concerning the meaning of eating and food to the various generations of this family. Then her mother asked if I could test the daughter's urine. I did, and it showed she had undiagnosed diabetes.

Conversations with the family present

People working in health and social care have one tremendous advantage from the point of view of exploring family stories. Family members, in their twos and threes, will often attend as a matter of routine: as couples, as parents with young children, or as children with old parents. These natural combinations do not need convening – they just happen. There are many occasions when some sort of family conversation is therefore not only possible, but a matter of courtesy. All the practitioner needs to do is to notice these occasions, and exploit the opportunities they provide for new narratives. Everyone who is present during a conversation is in effect a participant, even if their "'problem'" is that they are concerned about the identified client. The family member or neighbour who has apparently only been co-opted as a driver, or to assist with walking, is sometimes the person who, with encouragement, will volunteer the most useful information. In care homes and community centres, relatives who are present may be able to do the same, provided the person agrees.

In almost any circumstances, it may be worthwhile inviting patients and clients to bring their partners, friends, or neighbours on another occasion if they want to, explaining how helpful it is to have somebody else there to give another perspective. It can be surprising who people choose to bring with them: a sister rather than a spouse, a neighbour of the same age rather than an adult child, someone from the church or other place of worship rather than from the family. Inevitably, some will say no to the invitation, and this has to be respected. Equally, practitioners need to be aware that certain people might feel pressurised to have another person present against their wishes, and that in circumstances such as domestic violence this can carry significant danger. For that reason, it is often useful to request a one-to-one meeting at some point in the conversation, as well as involving others for part of it.

Does such an approach lead to an overwhelming increase in workload? Often, the reverse is the case. This is usually because it is possible to elicit a clearer story as a result, or because there are more human resources for exploring a new one. Many experienced practitioners report that they find it easier and more productive to work with couples or larger numbers of people in the consultation than with individuals, because of the energy and the range of possibilities for new stories that this produces. With more than two people in the room, there is a greater potential for asking questions about different perceptions, beliefs, theories, or suggestions for treatment or for change (Rivett and Street, 2009)

However, it is also worth sounding some cautions about inviting whole families to attend together. Although such invitations are standard practice in family therapy, they can also turn out to be unhelpful. Practical factors (small rooms, too little time, inadequate materials for toddlers, nervousness about having enough skill) may spoil the encounter unless there is a lot of thought beforehand. It also goes against what patients and clients may expect, so it may introduce an unnecessarily formal tone. Certainly, convening a whole-family meeting is a very powerful intervention, and should be offered with care: by a well-prepared practitioner, to a suitable person, at the right time, possibly with some kind of professional support such as an observer or supervisor – and never without prior discussion and informed consent.

Involving the family in the conversation

Sometimes people turn up to an encounter in health and social care in twos or threes because there is "a family problem," but usually this is not the case. They have come because of an identified problem in one individual, and want to express their views or offer help. They certainly do not want to go away feeling that they have a problem themselves, or are part of the problem.

One way of including whoever is present is by the technique that family therapists describe as "joining" a family. This means adopting the systematic habit of greeting everyone who arrives at the start of the consultation, finding out their identity and clarifying why they have come, unless it is perfectly obvious. By doing this, you can avoid discovering at the end of a consultation that the silent onlooker is deeply concerned about the person and actually has a lot to say or ask. Making eye contact with everyone in the room at regular intervals is another way of indicating a willingness to hear everyone. It may encourage everyone to be forthcoming without any further prompting.

Although "joining the family" sounds, and is, relatively simple, and many practitioners do so instinctively, some report that they have trouble doing it because of habits acquired in the past. These habits include focusing on the individual with the problem, while regarding everyone else as a kind of audience. However, once you have acquired the discipline of involving everyone in the conversation, you may be surprised by the people who speak up. This can include those with learning disabilities, toddlers, elderly people affected by dementia, and people whose English is poor that usually bring someone to speak on their behalf. Practitioners can also be surprised by the variety of perspectives that can be present at the same time, and the range of different stories that can come out as a result, or turning individual consultations into joint ones. For example, relatives are commonly bolder at speaking about the unexpressed fears of another family member, and may be more direct as advocates when there is dissatisfaction.

Generally, family members are very keen, and very relieved, when those accompanying them are brought into the orbit of the conversation, but sometimes they are not. They may even feel at risk of being upstaged. If this seems a possibility, it is important to ask permission before moving from a one-to-one dialogue into a wider conversation, for example by saying "Would you mind if I asked your daughter's view?" or "I'd find it helpful to hear what your wife has noticed. Is it

OK if I ask her?" Such strategies allow the possibility of other descriptions of the problem, and other suggestions for dealing with it. They also make it possible to help with a variety of different stories at the same time, for example a story of the worried relative along with the patient's story, as this case example shows.

Case example: Eric R

A practitioner gave this account:

> I have been seeing Eric R and his mother. The mother is now 84. The son is now 49, has a learning disability and has not worked since being made redundant from his job as a shop assistant a few years ago. They live together in a large house and have always seemed to have a close and protective relationship. They had a dog they adored, who died last year. A few months ago, the son started to complain of episodes of "spasms" in his throat. He described the sensation as feeling as if someone had their hands round his throat. He saw a hospital specialist, who found everything was normal. Then he saw a speech therapist to learn relaxation techniques. The spasms continued and got worse.
>
> When I saw him on a home visit, he said he wasn't depressed or worried about anything. His mother expressed concern about these symptoms as similar symptoms in the son's early twenties had resulted in several years of dependency on Valium. I felt I needed to know more about their life, so I listened while the mother talked. She told me how when the patient was 5, his father came home after being in prison for several years. Eric had no previous memories of him. The next day, they went out and the father became angry with the child as he would not sit the way he wanted him to. He shook his son violently. The boy was terrified and unable to breathe. This turned out to be the start of asthma.
>
> From the way she told this story, it was obvious it had been told many times over the years and was a very significant family story to them. The son was diagnosed as having "severe nervous asthma" and was taken to see many doctors, both NHS and private, during his childhood. The father was frequently violent towards the mother, but it was not until about 10 years later, after he had broken her collar bone, that the husband finally left. The mother told everyone this was for financial reasons. It is striking how much effect this man, who they have not seen for many years and is probably now dead, still has on their lives.
>
> On my next visit, I asked the mother some questions about the son's illness. I asked her what she thought his current spasms were caused by.

She said she thought he had been depressed since the death of the dog a few months ago. The son accepted this idea. He had always denied being worried about his mother's health, so I asked the mother if she thought Eric worried about her. She replied that he did, but it was not necessary, and she had told him not to worry. I said that maybe it was unrealistic for him not to worry given the mother's health problems, and maybe he should be allowed to worry. I also suggested that sometimes it was as difficult to watch someone being ill as to be ill oneself.

I subsequently saw Eric on his own. Over the next few weeks, the throat spasms resolved and he no longer seems depressed. The mother also seems happier, with fewer physical symptoms. My hypothesis was that the death of the dog reminded him that one day his mother will die and he will have to cope with life on his own.

Conversations with children

One dimension of family conversations requires specific attention. Children are present in many conversations, whether or not they are the reason for the encounter. Many professionals have had no special training in how to engage children in conversations. Unless they have children themselves, they may lack confidence in doing so. Although they may know quite a lot theoretically about child development, they may have little idea of the appropriate language and cognitive ability to expect of a child at any particular age. In addition, because the emphasis of training is so often on assessment rather than the narrative encounter, many practitioners may assume that it is enough to talk to parents *about* their children's experiences rather than to find out about these from the children themselves.

Fortunately, children are good teachers. Unlike adults, they will indicate that they have not understood a question by shrugging or looking blank rather than confabulating. This kind of feedback is a good way of learning whether questions make sense or not. Most children, especially young ones, tolerate fewer questions than adults. On the other hand, making it a principle to ask questions of children in every consultation when they are present (even if the identified patient in the consultation is a parent) will prevent them being bored and impatient. Any child in the room with any level of verbal ability is a person in his or her own right – and of course, one can still communicate with pre-verbal children in other ways.

From a narrative point of view, the child too has a story to tell. It may be a naive story, but it may be all the more honest, vivid and telling because of that. It may contain important information, perhaps by its very contrast from the adult's account. If a practitioner is confident and fluent in engaging children in conversation, and has taken the trouble to cultivate this skill, it will provide a good model for parents who want to develop this ability in themselves in order to give their children a clearer voice. Direct conversations with children can also be therapeutic for the children themselves, particularly if they feel as if they have had a chance to put their symptoms and worries into their own words, and if their anxieties can be allayed by face-to-face reassurance and explanations, so that they can take away a better story than the one brought into the surgery.

Conversations about family problems

Families do not speak with one voice. They have many. On most occasions, these voices support or complement each other, but there are also times when they are in discord. This may be apparent from the outset, because they have intentionally come to discuss a relationship problem. On other occasions, the discord becomes apparent as disagreements emerge during the conversation itself. The initial story may have been about something such as a medical problem, or depression, or a child's behaviour, but it then turns it into something else: explicit family conflict.

In dealing with family problems, some of the "seven C's" can be particularly helpful. An attitude of *curiosity* conveys that there is no "right" or "wrong" version of the story, and that the role of the professional is not to adjudicate or choose among competing versions. This in turn indicates to the family that the conversation is a safe space for expressing differences, and for exploring whether an agreed new narrative is possible. Again, *caution* is necessary here, since not every conversation is safe, especially if abuse or violence may be part of the picture.

Another mainstay of conversations with families is the use of *circularity*. Using circularity in this context involves several related techniques:

- Allowing everyone an opportunity to speak, by inviting all their views and moving between them as equitably as possible.
- Indicating a belief that everyone has a continuous effect on everyone else, so that it is unproductive to try to determine "who started it."
- Following a mode of questioning that invites others to move away from blaming and towards observing reciprocal effects and patterns.

One of the most helpful aspects of circularity is that it transmits the idea that there may not be a single solution to the family's difficulties, but at least there is an evolving conversation, and therefore the possibility of changing the story. Even if the new story does not emerge in the consultation itself, the conversation has provided a model for how old stories become unglued and new stories are created, as in the next case example.

Case example: Leo and Briony

A practitioner reported:

Leo came to see me asking if he could discuss his girlfriend's problem with me. He said she was no longer interested in sex with him for the last nine months but would push him away and burst into tears. I was curious that he was presenting "her" problem. I asked him what his girlfriend would say was wrong if she were there. He said "She just says she doesn't know, but she is very worried that she will lose me." We discussed his worries that she was upset with him and his frustration that this problem was persisting despite his sympathetic attitude. I suggested they return as a couple to see me.

Leo returned together with his girlfriend Briony. They sat close to each other holding hands. Briony said that her worst fear was the end of the relationship – they were each other's first sexual partners, and their only ones until he had been unfaithful. He explained it had "only been a one-night stand," and that he had immediately telephoned Briony, who was visiting her parents, to tell her and apologise. I asked about her reaction – she had been devastated and nearly decided not to come back from her parents, but he called so often that she came back to rejoin him. Their sexual relationship initially continued as normal and then the problems began. I asked how she reacted at the time. They agreed she had been very angry initially but expressed it very calmly, which was usual for her.

I asked her if she was still angry or upset about his unfaithfulness, and she said yes, she thought of it all the time. Leo then burst out in frustration, "I've told you I'll never do it again and I'm sorry, what else can I do?" The couple seemed stuck in this painful state, but terrified of separating. I shared these thoughts with them. I'm not experienced in this kind of conversation, and I wasn't sure it had any effect, but when I happened to see Briony a few weeks later, she said that it had made a big difference to both of them to be able to share what had happened in front of someone who didn't take sides and wasn't judgemental of either of them.

Different practitioners vary a great deal in how keen they are to tackle couple or family problems of this level of sensitivity in their everyday work. Some have been attracted to their jobs, and to further training, precisely because that is one of their interests. Others feel that they cannot offer the time or the skills to do this kind of work – and yet they recognise that it comes to them willy-nilly. Many families come to apparently "inappropriate" agencies to seek help because they see it as stigmatising to go somewhere else, or to accept an onward referral. For better or worse, just about any place in the health and social care sectors can become "de facto" somewhere that family therapy actually happens. Brief work of the kind described in the last case example may achieve more than many practitioners might expect, and certainly more than an onward referral that the family is unlikely to attend. While staying within the limits of their own interviewing skills and confidence, most practitioners seem to find it possible to extend their experience of such work, and then find it unexpectedly gratifying. Those who go on to acquire some degree of training in this work generally report that it becomes a cornerstone in their way of practising.Suggested exercises

1 In a series of consultations, ask for some basic information about "Who's at home?" What difference does this make to the rest of those consultations?
2 Choose one encounter when you are not too busy and where it seems appropriate to write down a more detailed genogram. What light does it shed on the problem and what effect does it have on the story?
3 Select two or three other ideas from this chapter (for example, "joining," asking children's views, asking questions of each family member in turn). How well does this fit with your normal practice? What effect does it have?
4 Start to experiment with using narrative questions when there is more than one person present. Which ones seem to work and which do not?

References

Asen, E., Tomson, D., Young, V. and Tomson, P. (2003) *Ten Minutes for the Family: Systemic Interventions in Primary Care*. London: Routledge.

Rivett, M. and Street, E. (2009) *Family Therapy: 100 Key Points and Techniques*. London: Routledge.

CHAPTER SEVEN

Mental health

Key ideas in this chapter

- Narrative ideas may provide a particularly useful framework for working with problems in the area of mental health.
- Narrative inquiry can be integrated with conventional psychological or psychiatric diagnosis and treatment.
- By working with narratives, practitioners in health and social care may be able to offer therapeutic input in a range of contexts, including family work and crisis intervention.

Introduction

Many practitioners in health and social care have reservations about the dominant ways of thinking about mental health problems. They are concerned that labels including "depression" or "post-traumatic stress disorder" can pathologise many people who are simply grappling with adverse life experiences (Heath, 1999; Summerfield, 2001; Frances, 2013; Greenberg, 2013; Grant, 2015). They also feel that labels generally offer a poor fit with the complex and ambiguous ways in which people present outside formal mental health settings.

By contrast, a narrative approach to mental health looks for accounts that primarily have meaning for the person, rather than labels that will satisfy the specialist. Although labels such as "depression" might be useful in some instances, including more severe forms of mental distress, narrative practitioners are more interested in finding a story that fits the uniqueness of what each person is going through. This is not an evasion of responsibility. It is a recognition that what matters most is whether the words make sense to the patient, rather than whether someone can be persuaded to accept a certain official designation. A diagnosis can then in effect take the form of a whole narrative rather than a single label (Launer, 2012). The following sections address different aspects of mental health, once again using examples from practitioners who have applied a narrative-based approach in their everyday work in health and social care.

Depression

Conventionally, health and social care professionals are trained to "detect depression" by asking specific questions about the patient's experience – for example, early morning waking, weight loss, and suicidal thoughts. Such questions certainly establish whether the client's description measures up to the agreed professional notion of depression. That in itself may be useful. It may help some patients and clients who want to try to locate their experiences along the spectrum of others' experiences, or who find it useful to have a name for what they are going through. It may also reassure professionals who want to make sure that they are not forgetting to inquire about important indicators of personal risk. However, there are obvious problems too. A diagnosis can in itself be a form of amplifying and prolonging the problem. A focus on defining and concretising symptoms may also distract practitioners from trying to make fuller sense of others' experiences, or exploring their clients' preferred options for change.

An alternative narrative framework for talking with people who appear to be depressed involves offering them the label of depression without insisting that it has to be relevant or useful. There are questions such as:

- "What words would you use to describe these feelings?"
- "What do you think has brought them about, or contributed to them?"
- "Some people would use the word 'depression' to describe what you are going through – how useful would you find that in your own case?"

Such questioning offers patients the landmark of a recognised term if that is what they wish, without closing down dialogue or stigmatising them if it is not how they view their problems. Either way, it does not presuppose a particular form of intervention, since it leaves open the option of saying at a later stage in the consultation:

- "Are there particular kinds of help you want to consider?"
- "What are your thoughts about medication?"

The point of such inquiries is not to nudge others towards the practitioner's preferred form of treatment. It is to keep alive a sense of negotiability about symptoms, choices, and the way forward. It also maintains the professional's usefulness in the many instances where patients do not want to conceptualise their experiences simply in the way that the health and social care professions find most convenient. It leaves open the possibility of alternative approaches such as looking at the person's family background with the aid of a genogram, or suggesting that a partner or close relative might come along in order to give a wider understanding of what is going on. Most importantly, it lets clients enter into dialogue about how they prefer to define their story. That can certainly include medical, psychological or psychiatric ways of conceptualising the world, and many people appear to be happy to choose that way for themselves. However, a narrative approach is one that does not summarily close down other ways of understanding personal turmoil and distress.

It is of course important to acknowledge the limits to a narrative approach of this kind. Faced with a patient with incapacitating or life-threatening patterns of thought and behaviour, or significant cognitive impairment, it can occasionally be dangerous to pursue such inquiry. However, the uncommon occurrence of extreme risks seems to constrain many professionals from taking a more liberating approach in the generality of cases. Far more often, it is possible to give permission to patients and clients to take a more biographical approach to their experiences, and to discuss their symptoms at the same time as addressing issues from their work, home life and family background. This can lead to the discovery of a middle ground where no one is minimising the degree of their suffering, nor are their problems being reduced to a single-word definition. This kind of biographical approach to someone feeling depressed is illustrated by the following example.

Case example: Meryem H

A practitioner told this story:

Meryem H is about 50, and has a diagnosis of long-standing depression. I always used to get bogged down with her. She has had four children, a boy of 19 who had left home three months ago to live by himself, another who would have been 21 but died in a swimming accident three years ago at the age of 18, and two girls in their mid-teens who were still living at home. She has divorced her husband. I realised I did not know her very well apart from the bare bones of her story, and I wanted to start from scratch. I decided to set aside time to try to get to know her better.

When she came, she told me she has been increasingly depressed since the death of her oldest son. She talked about the guilt she felt if she did anything that began to feel as if she was enjoying herself, so she spent most of her time lying in bed blaming herself for past events, and visiting her son's grave. She was aware that her other children wanted her to do things like going shopping with her daughters, or going out to buy her surviving son new clothes. She felt unable to do this because she thought of her dead son all the time and she would end up crying if she went out with her other children. This made her feel guilty, and she knew that they felt resentful of the dead brother who appeared to be her favourite child.

She also felt guilty because she had known for many years that her marriage was not working. She feels that if she had split up with her husband years before, then perhaps her son would not have died. As her other son approached the age at which his brother had died, she was worried that something might happen to him too. She had tried to stop him moving away from home, and when he came round for meals now she would often cry and her son would hug her.

I felt that it was important to acknowledge the sadness of her story. I pointed out to her that she had managed to continue to be a good mother to her children and that they obviously wanted to spend time in her company even though one had left home. She was visibly moved by this statement. Her whole body language changed. She sat up and leaned forward in her chair to hear what was next. I took the risk of being quite directive and suggesting that she set aside a period of time each week for each of her children and devote that time to them individually to doing whatever each of them wished to do in that time.

I now see her at intervals of three or four weeks to see how she is getting on with this. The approach seems to have worked. She does sometimes talk about her depression, but far less. Mainly, we just talk about her life, which now seems to be going somewhere, though slowly.

Psychosis

People who experience psychotic thinking bring unusual and peculiar stories to health and social care professionals. From the point of view of taking a narrative-based approach, there is a risk that professionals might be drawn into delusional ideas to the point of accepting them as true. There are indeed practitioners who have advocated this within the worlds of psychiatry and of family therapy (Anderson and Goolishian, 1992). However, there are two good reasons for not going to this extreme in the majority of health and social care settings:

- Most practitioners work within professional networks where such a relativistic approach would still generally be seen as unethical and destructive.
- It might prevent professionals from noticing serious risk.

Set against this, however, there is the far commoner risk that professionals can discount anything clients say as evidence of disordered thinking, and therefore not worthy of any exploration. This effectively deprives such people of the sort of conversation that takes place with every other patient, and is unjust. Professionals in many fields are nowadays seeing it as increasingly important to provide good all-round care to those who have been given the diagnosis of schizophrenia or paranoia, rather than just focusing on their mental state. It may be equally important to see that they are included within the orbit of normal and respectful conversations as much as anyone else. A narrative approach can help to ensure that clients have a sense of being included as active participants in their own well-being, however unusual their perceptions and experiences may be.

In practice, it is perfectly possible to hold conversations with psychotic patients that hover on the razor's edge in this respect. This means accepting their language in the context of the conversation, while not letting go of one's perception of them as disturbed, distressed and in need of protection. For example, it may be better to use ambiguous wording such as "How long do you think people in the street have been talking about you?" rather than "How long have you been imagining that people are talking about you?" Such an approach has the advantage that one can enter the linguistic world of the patient without surrendering a hold on one's own view of reality. Working in this way, on the borderline between rejection of the story and collusion with it, appears to enhance trust and increase the possibility of having thoughtful conversations about things such as medication.

Case example: Ben T

A practitioner said:

> I see a man with schizophrenia called Ben T regularly. He always talks about people on "death row" in America. He says he writes them letters but I don't know how far that is true. Sometimes he cries when he talks about them. I think in a way he is talking about his own suffering, but I don't think he would understand if I confronted him with this. Instead, I usually tell him that I regard his concern as a sign of his sensitivity to the suffering of others. We talk about the death row convicts a lot, and in a sense I suppose I am using it as a metaphor for him, but I don't think that really matters.

Crisis intervention

When workers in health and social care see individuals or families in crisis, the response is often to make a referral to a counsellor, psychologist or psychiatrist.

However, by the time these appointments arrive, the crisis may have "gone off the boil." The emotional impetus for change has been lost, and the home situation may have solidified around an intractable symptom or a sense of fatalism. By the same token, there are opportunities for crisis intervention using a narrative-based approach in ordinary health and social care settings that barely exist elsewhere. The next case example gives an account of one such intervention.

Case example: Mary W

A practitioner told this story:

> Mary is 17. Her parents divorced when she was 3. Her mother subsequently remarried and had two further children, a boy now aged 8 and a girl of 5.
>
> Two months ago, just a week before Christmas, Mary took an overdose. She had spent three days in a local hospital being washed out and monitored. Mary said initially that the overdose was because of a row with her boyfriend over the amount of time they spent together. Mary had promised she would not do it again.
>
> When I saw her, Mary asked if her mother could be with her in her consultation. Mary began the consultation crying. She said she had recently moved away from the family home to live with her boyfriend. The boyfriend works night shifts as a baker. She finds the long evenings alone frightening, and quite different from what she expected. Her loneliness was worse because recently her mother and stepfather sold the old family home and moved with their two young children some distance away.
>
> Mary then really started to reproach her mother, in front of me. She accused her mother of spending less time with her in recent months. Then she began to complain how little she had been allowed to see her real father during her upbringing. It emerged that she had only met him five times after her parents' separation when she was 18 months old. He died from a heart attack when she was 14. She talked of how she had been forced to accept her stepfather, and his surname, and of how she had always felt jealous of her half-brother and half-sister, and less valued than them.
>
> Her mother seemed to want to explain to me the facts of the situation as she saw it. I asked her to talk about what it had been like as a single mother. She told me she had been deserted by Mary's father. Before that, her husband used to spend most of his time and nearly all their money in betting shops. She explained that after the separation, he rarely used his right to have contact with his daughter. She also said that, to her mind, her present husband could not have been more thoughtful about Mary's upbringing.

I tried to move the conversation on. I asked them to compare their different versions. I used questions like "Do you see things the same way as Mary on this issue?" and "Would you like to comment on what your mother has just said?" For a long stretch of time, I just sat as a sort of a referee while they explained, argued, protested and just listened to each other.

At that point, I gave them a description of the problem as I saw it. I talked about Mary's loneliness. I noted her disappointment at her new life, and the various changes in her circumstances. I offered a suggestion that she was having a delayed grieving. I wondered if selling the family home might seem like the final burial of all her hopes about being part of an ideal family. I also told Mrs W that I appreciated how hard her role was. She had wanted to support Mary through the bereavement. But she wanted her own past hardship and effort to be acknowledged.

I saw them again a week later. Mary came into the room relaxed and smiling. They explained what had passed between them. Mrs W had been able to talk about how her first husband abandoned them after years of violence, coercive control and emotional abuse. Mary had managed to engage with this. She had also realised how angry and betrayed she felt herself.

I also did some troubleshooting. I asked them what they expected would be the next turning points, or changes, in Mary's life. She talked about her boyfriend and the possibility of marriage, but she wasn't sure about that. She said that if he had more confidence, he would consider retraining so he could take a job that gave him more time with her. I trod really delicately here, because he wasn't in the room, but I did say I would be very happy to see him and Mary together if they wished.

Frequent service users

Almost every professional will be aware of users who make repeated demands on services, or bring the same unchanging lament on each occasion. They are sometimes discussed under the disparaging label of "heartsink patients" (Moscrop, 2011). Interestingly, people who make one practitioner's heart sink can often leave others' hearts quite unaffected. It might therefore be more appropriate to talk of "heartsink interactions." It is worth speculating how professionals might alter their view of the matter by considering which clients and families have the opposite effect: one might call these "heartleap patients."

In the case of any negative interaction, it can help to consider the following questions:

- What purpose do frequent demands or repeated laments serve? How might these be addressed by asking new questions, or exploring alternative accounts of what is going on?
- What are the client's contexts that are being ignored? Does a repetitive story become more negotiable if more is known about the person's genogram, current household or working circumstances?
- Does the client feel as stuck as the practitioner – or is there something comforting in the very repetitiveness of the story?
- Does the professional's inability to ask any new questions reflect the limitations of the working context (e.g. if I ask this question and she gives that answer, I still don't have anywhere I can send her)?
- What questions could the professional ask that might challenge someone to describe their experiences in a different way?
- What questions might revive the practitioner's own curiosity and help them to see the person not as annoying and burdensome, but as someone unique, interesting and worthy of compassion?

Questions that seem useful in these kinds of interactions are often very broad ones, and also simple:

- "What's the best thing going on in your life at the moment?"
- "Are there things in your life that you've never told me about, but might help me understand you better?"
- "I'm curious to know what keeps you coming back when your visits here often don't seem to make anything better for you."
- "I wanted to ask you how you view our consultations, and what you get out of them?"

It would be idealistic to say that questions such as these always turn repetitive interactions into sparklingly refreshing ones, but they do often yield surprising results, especially revelations from the patients that they have derived support and benefit from consultations that the professional has felt were going nowhere. An equally common outcome is for the practitioner to say "Until I'd asked that question and got an answer, I never really understood the person. Now, I feel I do." Inevitably, some interactions do continue like video loops, in spite of the most imaginative efforts – but trying and failing to elicit a new story still makes the practitioner feel better than never having tried. It may also uncover the fact that frequent conversations about stuck problems are the "least worst": they may be preferable, for example, to complete isolation or to suicide.

Perhaps the most impressive analysis ever written about a family of frequent consulters appears in a paper by the GP Christopher Dowrick with the appealing title "Why do the O'Sheas consult so often?" Dowrick showed how he and his colleagues attempted to work with a family of frequent consulters bringing complex needs to his GP surgery. The team used a variety of tools to approach this work, including hypothesis generation, hypothesis testing, and strategising. However, the core database for the work was a combination of the family genogram coupled with information about the consultation rates of the various members. One striking correlation that emerged from this was between consulting behaviour and the loss of significant people – including doctors in the practice who had retired (Dowrick, 1992).

Somatisation and "medically unexplained symptoms"

There is an extensive literature about patients who experience undiagnosable physical ailments, or conditions where the exact cause has become the focus of heated controversy. Much of the literature addresses ways in which such people might be influenced to talk about psychosocial issues in their lives rather than dwelling on physical symptoms (Smith et al., 2006; Hatcher and Arroll, 2008). Common experience certainly suggests that there is often more possibility of movement and of helpful understanding when patients can frame problems in terms of the difficulties they face in their lives, rather than simply their subjective experience of malfunction in their bodies. However, in helping others construct new and more effective stories about what is happening to them, it is usually useful to remain neutral in relation to their understanding of themselves. It is worth remembering that we live in a culture where physical symptoms are often seen as more legitimate than emotional difficulties, and where many people tend to tell stories of their distress in terms of somatic perceptions rather than mental manifestations. In addition, professionals too may have shown more interest in their physical symptoms than anything else, thus amplifying them further. A very important role for professionals may therefore be to regard these problems instead as "medically unexplored stories" with more curiosity than challenge, and with an acceptance that the professional's construction of the problem may need to be regarded as no more privileged than the client's (Kirmayer, 2004; Launer, 2009).

The following principles seem to help in this challenging area:

- It is counterproductive to challenge, either overtly or subtly, people's own stories about their symptoms. Until they feel that that professionals have adequately heard their story of having an undiagnosed tumour, or intractable chronic fatigue, they are unlikely to be willing to frame their experiences in any other way.

- If professionals are hoping for more flexibility from patients in regard to their symptoms, it is also appropriate to hold on to the possibility that patients might turn out to be entirely right in their own assessment of their condition.
- It is often helpful to share the dilemma of making multiple investigations and referrals with the patients concerned. For example, it is possible to say "I can order another X-ray if that's what you want, but can we also start to think about what we're going to do if everything turns out to be normal again . . . ?"
- Taking a genogram or inquiring into the family background can be done in a way that does not imply any blame or responsibility, but may reveal a great deal and move the patient's preoccupation away from pain and suffering.

Suggested exercises

1 Think of a recent professional encounter with someone who has a psychiatric diagnosis such as depression. What does the diagnosis offer them, and what does it withhold from them?
2 Think of someone whose narrative often seems repetitive or "stuck." Make a list of questions you have never asked that person that might take the conversation in a new direction next time.
3 What resources are available to you in response to a mental health crisis? Are there ways that you might consider extending your involvement in these kinds of crises? What would make it possible to do so safely?

References

Anderson, H. and Goolishian, H. (1992) The client is the expert: a not-knowing approach to therapy. In S. McNamee and K. Gergen (eds), *Therapy as Social Construction*. London: Sage, pp. 25–39.

Dowrick, C. (1992) Why do the O'Sheas consult so often? An exploration of complex family illness behaviour. *Social Science and Medicine*, 34, 491–497.

Frances, A. (2013) *Saving Normal: An Insider's Revolt Against Out-of-Control Psychiatric Diagnosis, DSM-5, Big Pharma, and the Medicalization of Ordinary Life*. New York: William Morrow.

Grant, A. (2015) Demedicalising misery: welcoming the human paradigm in mental health nurse education. *Nurse Education Today*, 35, e50–e53.

Greenberg, G. (2013) *The Book of Woe: The DSM and the Unmaking of Psychiatry*. New York: Blue Rider Press.

Hatcher, S. and Arroll, B. (2008) Assessment and management of medically unexplained symptoms. *BMJ*, 336, 1124–1128.

Heath, I. (1999) Commentary: there must be limits to the medicalization of human distress. *BMJ*, 318, 440.

Kirmayer, L. (2004) Explaining medically unexplained symptoms. *Canadian Journal of Psychiatry*, 49, 663–672.

Launer, J. (2009) Medically unexplored stories. *Postgraduate Medical Journal*, 85, 503–504.

Launer, J. (2012) Narrative diagnosis. *Postgraduate Medical Journal*, 88, 115–116.

Moscrop, A. (2011) "Heartsink" patients in general practice: a defining paper, its impact, and psychodynamic potential. *British Journal of General Practice*, 61(586), 346–348.

Smith, R.C., Lyles, J.S., Gardiner, J.C., Sirbu, C., Hodges, A., Collins, C., et al. (2006) Primary care clinicians treat patients with medically unexplained symptoms: a randomized controlled trial. *Journal of General Internal Medicine*, 21, 671–677.

Summerfield, D. (2001) The invention of post-traumatic stress disorder and the social usefulness of a psychiatric category. *BMJ*, 322, 95–98.

CHAPTER EIGHT

Supervision

Key ideas in this chapter

- In complex and demanding fields such as health and social care, many professionals feel they might benefit from regular reflective supervision, but comparatively few receive it.
- When practitioners help each other to think about their work, it can improve care. It can also help them to develop their overall skills in questioning and reflection.
- Narrative concepts and techniques work just as well in supervision as in direct care.
- Narrative inquiry can be combined with advice and guidance, just as it can in work with clients.
- Practitioners can learn how to carry out better supervision with their colleagues, informally as well as formally, and in either one-to-one or group encounters.

Introduction

All the chapters so far have focused on one kind of encounter – the encounter between a practitioner and service users. This chapter looks at how to apply a narrative-based approach to supervising other professionals, whether they are peers or learners. Narrative-based supervision has a ready-made methodology, since the ideas of curiosity, complexity and so forth, and techniques such as hypothesising and questioning, can be applied in supervising other professionals just as they can in conversations with clients (Whiting, 2007; Halpern and Morrison, 2012; Launer, 2013). Indeed, as the introduction to this book explained, it may be easier to begin by learning "Conversations Inviting Change" in the context of peer supervision before practising it in one's other work.

Within health and social care, opportunities for supervision vary greatly according to the particular traditions and requirements of each discipline. In some professions, such as counselling, it occurs as part of routine professional work. In others, such as medicine, it may only take place in the context of training, management or remediation – or does not happen at all. Supervision also comes in many different forms. It can occur one-to-one or in groups, formally or informally, and between peers or in a hierarchical relationship. The boundaries between supervision and other activities such as coaching and mentoring are sometimes unclear, but definitions are probably less important than understanding the context and purpose of any encounter (Proctor, 2010). Because of this, the following list of questions can be helpful for both supervisors and supervisees to consider in order to put their conversations in context (Clark et al., 2006):

- Who is asking for this conversation to happen?
- What do they want, and why?
- Do they know what the supervisor can and cannot offer?
- Is the supervisee attending voluntarily?
- Is anyone expecting specific outcomes, should they be, and if so, what?
- Who, if anyone, is paying whom, and do all the parties know this?
- Who is reporting to whom, about what, exactly when, and do all the parties know this?
- Is everyone agreed on the terms being used, and on their meaning?

Whatever the profession or the context, professionals who carry out supervision often have to manage a subtle and fluctuating relationship between "looking over someone's shoulder" and in the different sense of "looking after someone." We sometimes symbolise this dual task using the diagram shown in Figure 8.1. The left-hand circle denotes supervision as a top-down activity, and represents the duty of supervisors to give clear instruction and maintain standards. The right-hand circle, using the words "Super" and "Vision," represents their responsibility to inspire supervisees to develop their professional identity and autonomy.

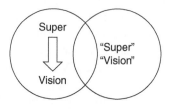

Figure 8.1   The two faces of supervision: instruction and inspiration

We have found the following key principles useful in teaching and applying narrative-based supervision. The examples are taken from practitioners who have applied a narrative-based approach when supervising others.

Case presentations are narratives

If service users bring stories that are tentative, incomplete, or confused, this is also true of practitioners who report on cases that are puzzling or upsetting them. The same disjunctions and hesitancy, repetitiveness and vagueness, characterise both. Supervision using a narrative-based approach offers practitioners the same facility that narrative-based practice offers to clients. This is the opportunity to present a story and have someone interrogate it intelligently and sensitively, so there is the possibility of a new story. Interestingly, there is often a "parallel process" between helping the practitioner with a new story and helping the client with one. In other words, practitioners who carry out their work with a more coherent sense of what is going on and what possibilities there might be for moving the story forward are far more likely to help the colleagues and students they see to create more satisfactory new narratives. The benefits of this process even extend more widely – to more imaginative conversations generally.

Even if the relationship between the supervisor and supervisee is that of a senior to a junior, a narrative-based stance will both facilitate the presentation of the case as well as demonstrating how this can be done with clients. By showing a capacity for holding onto uncertainty and avoiding inappropriate foreclosure, supervisors can model the same capacity for others. We have found that it often helps to start a conversation about a case by asking what the supervisee would like help with, or any particular kind of focus they would like their supervisor to have. Even when the answer is relatively vague (e.g. "I have the feeling I'm missing something important, but I'm not sure what"), it will often help if the supervisor can craft some questions to bring more focus to the conversation, rather than making unexamined assumptions about what the supervisee wants or needs. Similarly, it also helps to ask at the end what the supervisee got out of the session (if anything), what ideas have been most useful, which questions the supervisee would now like to ask the client at their next meeting, or which options seem the ones most likely to be worth pursuing clinically.

There is inevitably a place for advice and guidance in supervision, just as there is in all professional work. In some conversations, the supervisor has a legal or regulatory responsibility for the person being supervised, and this needs to be transparent. Some practitioners will genuinely have more experience of particular kinds of cases than their colleagues, and it would be inappropriate for them to withhold good ideas. However, there are a number of helpful guidelines that can protect supervisors from appearing too assertive or impeding the other person's narrative. One guideline is not to offer advice or suggestions too early in the supervision session. This helps to avoid closing down the conversation too soon and blocking off important opportunities for exploring the issues further. It is also often helpful to seek permission before offering advice (for example, with a question such as "How useful would it be at this moment if I suggested a possible way forward?"). Advice can also be repackaged within a series of graded questions to test the water and see if the colleague might find it helpful ("What do think would happen if you tried . . . ?"). The most important safeguard in this respect is to follow feedback from supervisees, and to notice when they want to continue explaining the difficulties of the case rather than receive advice – even if this may be necessary at some point for reasons of professional governance.

Because of the complexities of combining a managerial role with one that facilitates the evolution of a new narrative, it is also sometimes easier for a colleague from a completely different professional background, or without line management responsibility, to help another practitioner see a case in a new light, as the following case example shows.

Case example: a case of pain

A male gynaecologist on one of our courses brought a case for supervision involving a patient with a long history of pain for which no cause had ever been found. He was very unsure how to go forward with this woman, who consulted often. A female care home manager who was on the same training course agreed to interview the gynaecologist about the case. What became clear through her questioning was that the doctor felt sure the patient was depressed, but over several months had often got into very unproductive discussions with her over this, when she vehemently denied any depression or emotional problems of any sort. He had also offered her antidepressants a number of times to see if it would make a difference to her pain, but she had refused. He knew that she was married and did not seem to be very happy with her husband, and on one occasion he had asked her directly about her sex life, but said she was extremely reluctant to talk about this and seemed to think it irrelevant.

The course participant acting as peer supervisor widened the discussion to find out if there were areas of the patient's life that the doctor did not know about, or which he might be curious to inquire into. It also became clear that the overwhelming emphasis on symptoms and diagnosis had prevented him from asking about a wide range of other issues, including her work, her wider family, and her childhood – perhaps to a surprising extent, given the nature and chronicity of the symptoms. With the peer supervisor's help, he chose a number of areas he might explore to find out more about her, and move the consultations away from their usual "tramlines."

Returning to the next course day a fortnight later, the gynaecologist reported having had a very productive consultation with the woman. He discovered she had been made redundant as a teacher at about the time the pain started, and had been very disheartened at not being able to find another job. He also found out that she had been adopted as a child and was currently engaged in a search for her birth mother. He commented: "I don't know if any of this will turn out to be relevant, but I think it's probably the first consultation I've ever had with her when she didn't say 'Well what's causing it then?'"

Contexts are just as important as content

Professionals who feel "stuck" with cases are often preoccupied with the precise events of the case: who said what to whom and when, what happened and why, and what occurred as a result. Yet when a case is causing difficulty, it nearly always seems to be because there are misunderstandings or muddles in one of the surrounding contexts. It often turns out, for example, that difficulties have arisen in a case not because of any intrinsic complexity but because people in the professional network were in some way working at cross purposes without being aware of this. Or it might be that, in spite of an apparent familiarity with all the details of the case, the supervisee has never paused to think about the role they are playing themselves in the interaction.

For this reason, it is often useful at a very early stage to ask a question such as "What do I need to know about your work setting that may have a bearing on this?" or "Apart from you, who else is involved in this person's care?" Asking questions of this kind can prevent the conversation becoming bogged down early in excessive data, and help both parties to focus on more quickly on the crux, or potential crux, of the story. They may also draw attention to a possible contextual factor that had been paralysing the situation but had gone unnoticed. Clearly, there needs to be a balance between eliciting too much detail in a case and eliciting too little. A clinician who gets no chance to spell out the bare bones of the case is likely to feel deprived. On the other hand, going into great detail can waste valuable time, and prevent a different kind of story ever emerging. Box 8.1 gives an example of one GP providing effective (and remarkably brief) supervision to another GP colleague.

Box 8.1   A GP supervises a younger colleague

In this dialogue, an experienced GP called Angela is listening to Sarah, a younger colleague. Sarah has just given an account of a consultation she had the previous day. Her patient was a large, white middle-class, middle-aged man, whose wife is a doctor. He had come requesting a referral to a hospital on the instruction of his wife. Sarah had felt frustrated that this patient's wife seemed to be suggesting a hospital referral for something that could be managed in primary care, but felt that she was not able to respond to the patient in a way that would be most conducive to his health. She had written the referral for him and she did not think he had noticed her frustration, but wanted to discuss what to do the next time he came. Sarah's conversation with Angela continues as follows:

Sarah: I find this man so difficult, he waltzes in and always tells me what his wife wants me to organise. I don't always think these referrals are necessary, and I know I could manage him better in general practice if only he gave me the opportunity.

Angela: Is there anything else you think it would be useful for me to know about this issue?

Sarah: He works as a banker in a large successful organisation and his wife is a consultant microbiologist in a local hospital, and I feel intimidated by them.

Angela: Intimidated . . . can you tell me more about being intimidated?

Sarah: Yes, I always dread it when these powerful men like him come into the surgery and make demands of me. I feel that I have to follow what they want even if I don't feel that it's the best way to manage the problem.

Angela: If he was, for instance, an unemployed small woman, what difference do you think this would make to your interaction?

Sarah: Oh, that would be completely different . . . [Sarah went on to describe her medical management plan.]

Angela: If this patient and his wife were listening to this conversation now, what do you think they would say . . . ?

Sarah: I think they would be surprised by my feeling of powerlessness and I think they would possibly accept my management. I think that they are so used to hospital medicine that they don't really know about our expertise in primary care . . .

Angela's comments after the conversation:

Before I did narrative training, I would probably have offered advice early on about how to manage the patient next time ("Yes, I find this type of patient difficult too – why don't you try this . . . " type of suggestion). From this conversation, maybe Sarah reflected on the reasons for the consultation being difficult for her and had some space to think about the reasons she felt intimidated. It gave her an opportunity to consider how the patient and his wife view medical care from their positions, which perhaps freed her to introduce them to the expertise she offers from a primary care point of view.

(adapted from Miller, 2012)

Personal issues and feelings need delicate handling

Most practitioners have probably had the experience of seeing someone who reminded them of people in their own personal lives. They may also have got into difficulties with particular kinds of individuals who caused anxiety, anger and emotional over-involvement. In addition, most would probably have to confess that some clients have excited them sexually, while others have repelled them, made them feel very uncomfortable, or reduced them to tears. Such experiences cannot be ignored in case discussions, but they also need to be handled with delicacy, especially in a group or team context.

Because professionals supervising their colleagues on cases have an apparent licence to ask whatever they want, some are tempted to ask questions such as "Does this person remind you of your mother?" or "Do you find her sexually attractive?" or "Have you had an illness like this yourself in the past?" Most practitioners react with discomfort to such intrusiveness, feeling quite rightly that they have volunteered themselves for some support from a colleague and not for amateur psychotherapy. If a supervisor forms a hypothesis that personal issues are relevant, it is more respectful to ask a general question about the kind of territory involved without stepping into the territory itself. This means, for example, starting with a general question such as "When you think about this case, does it take you into an area that is quite difficult to talk about?" If the answer is yes, the supervisor can then seek permission to take a small step forward, for example by asking "Is it possible for you to say what the area is, or is that something you would rather keep to yourself for the time being?" An inquiry along these lines does sometimes open up the possibility of taking a gradual series of steps that makes it possible for the client to receive help even in a very emotion-laden case. At the same time, it is vital both for the supervisor and supervisee to keep the escape routes open. Case presenters need to know in advance that they are in the driving seat with regard to what they do and do not wish to disclose. They also need the assurance of their colleague that there will be total confidentiality regarding any disclosures.

Supervision is also not the only option for help in these circumstances. It may be quite appropriate to ask a practitioner "If it doesn't seem right to talk about this issue here and now, who else could you talk to about this?" Sometimes, the answer to this question is that there is another colleague whom the client can use as a resource in this way. It is also impossible to dodge the issue that some colleagues and trainees may show signs of being in considerable personal turmoil during a case supervision, or they will disclose that they are dealing with cases where they feel emotionally overwhelmed and out of their depth. Anyone offering supervision needs to be prepared to have an entirely private discussion of what help may be needed by the person concerned, including counselling or therapy. The supervision conversation might therefore need to be put on hold. Where appropriate, supervisors should also be equipped with knowledge of other resources, professional or psychological, to deal with a supervisee experiencing distress that goes far wider than their professional casework.

Case example: terminal care

A hospice chaplain brought a case to one of our workshops. It involved a man with advanced cancer. His son was insisting that no one should tell either of his parents the prognosis, and that everyone should just say that he was being treated for a big liver because some people got that in old age. The chaplain felt that this was quite wrong, and that patients normally guess what is happening anyway. She found it very hard to be tolerant of the son's view and felt inclined to override his wishes.

In a supervision interview with the course group as observers, it became clear that the chaplain's strong beliefs were very much influenced by personal experience, as her own mother had died from advanced cancer. She felt the health and social care workers involved had been very evasive with all her family and she had resolved never to do so with her own patients. At first, she found it difficult to talk about this in front of a course group and became tearful. The course tutor intervened to check with the chaplain if she wanted the interview to continue. She said she did as it was important to her to separate her own feelings and experiences from the needs of her job, and she thought the interviewer was being very sensitive. With considerable tact, the supervisor helped her to think of how to explore her patient's own experience or wishes. Quite a long way on in the interview, she admitted that the patient himself had never seemed to be very bothered or curious about his condition. She had never really had a conversation with the son about who else in the family did or didn't know the prognosis, and what he feared would happen if his father found out. The family were from a different culture, and she had not explored with them what would normally happen in their country of origin concerning the open discussion of a poor prognosis.

Good supervision takes time

Among counsellors and therapists, it is common for supervision on a single case to last for up to an hour. Given the normal working pace of health and social care, and the number of complex cases that may invite discussion, this can seem like a ridiculous luxury. However, there are a number of good reasons for setting aside reasonable periods of time for discussions with colleagues about a difficult case – probably not less than 15 or 20 minutes – whether in one-to-one supervision or in a group. It is also worth specifying in advance how long is available, so that those who bring cases can tailor their accounts accordingly.

First, the longer the discussion about a case lasts, the more chance there is that the person presenting it will change their story from a stuck and repetitive one to a different kind of story where new options have opened up. It is common to hear a colleague express pessimism for the first 10 or 15 minutes of presenting a case, but then gradually unfreeze and start to develop a new story. Similarly, interviewers may feel as hopelessly overwhelmed as the presenters to start with, but then gradually become more imaginative and flexible in their questioning. The experience of this process, on either side, introduces practitioners to the idea that any case offers multiple possibilities for different approaches, however stuck it might initially have seemed.

Another advantage of a long discussion about a case is that it gives the participants extended practice in conducting "Conversations Inviting Change," especially if they are new to this kind of questioning. They can practise forms of questioning that may be new to them, including inquiring into how a problem might appear from the perspective of the presenter's colleagues or others involved in the system. They can do this without too much time pressure and then transfer the techniques not only to shorter conversations with colleagues at work, but also to routine consultations with patients.

Perhaps the most important argument in favour of spending time on a case is that it promotes deep reflection generally, and therefore acts as a counter to the prevalent culture of telling anecdotes as the only way of communicating one's distress or difficulties with the work. This is not to deride anecdotes. They can fulfil an important function in helping professionals to offload their anxiety and stress levels, and perhaps even to seek some simple ideas of how to handle cases in different ways. However, they can also promote a "coffee room culture" that stereotypes patients and reinforces habits of stuckness. The exchange of anecdotes can also degenerate into a tit-for-tat competition in much the same way that people who go fishing proverbially boast about having caught a bigger fish than anyone else. By contrast, experience of prolonged case discussion can potentially influence the work setting so that reflective discussion becomes the norm instead. Although there are many settings where prolonged discussion of this kind may be an occasional luxury rather than a routine, each episode of reflection can lead to a boost in the clinician's ability to manage a difficult case, and perhaps the workload generally for a period of time.

In time, practitioners do acquire the ability to move faster in thinking about cases, either as supervisors or presenters. Familiarity with circular questioning, and repeated help with difficult cases, leads them to think better on their feet when discussing cases in the future. These activities build up their confidence in making effective interventions in group discussions – for example, by framing brief but highly pertinent questions. Such experience also appears to lead to a greater general optimism about cases that might otherwise appear intractable.

Case example: asking to see someone more senior

A drug worker in her twenties explained on one of our courses how a 50-year-old man had recently seen her for a consultation, but asked at the end of the consultation if he could see someone "more senior" for his next appointment. Her clinic's policy was not to do this unless the level of complexity of the case suggested it was necessary. She had tried to explain this to the man, but this had led to quite a hostile reaction and left her feeling very uncomfortable. He said he would come back for one more meeting but would expect to see someone more senior subsequently as he had some concerns that he felt only someone with more experience could deal with. A colleague on the course interviewed her and tried to establish what her beliefs were about her work and the drug clinic. She said she felt confident working with older people. She disliked onward referrals, and was afraid that colleagues would see any such cases as "failures" on her part. When the interviewer asked her about the client's beliefs, she explained he was "quite a middle-class sort of guy," and he probably believed that older professionals were more reliable than younger ones.

The supervisor then explored various scenarios with her, defining a spectrum from "confrontation" to "surrender." This helped the drug worker to define a middle position of compromise between these two. She decided she would be willing to refer the client onwards with good grace, but first wanted to have a wider discussion with him about his views. For example, what experiences had he had previously when seeking help? Also, was he willing to give her at least some headlines about the concerns he felt he could only disclose to an older person?

Suggested exercises

1 Next time a colleague wants to discuss a difficult case, offer to set aside some time for peer supervision, and use it to practise narrative interviewing.

2 When you need help on a difficult case yourself, ask a colleague to interview you about the case, explaining that you want to be questioned
   rather than advised.
3 When you are next taking part in a group discussion of a case, try to
   make all your interventions in the form of questions about the case rather
   than offering information or suggestions.

References

Clark, P., Jamieson, A., Launer, J., Trompetas, A., Whiteman, J. and Williamson, D. (2006) Intending to be a supervisor, mentor or coach: which, what for and why? *Education for Primary Care*, 17, 109–116.

Halpern, H. and Morrison, S. (2012) Narrative-based supervision. In D. Owen and R. Shohet (eds), *Clinical Supervision in the Medical Profession: Structured Reflective Practice.* Maidenhead: Open University Press, pp. 73–81.

Launer, J. (2013) Narrative-based supervision. In L.S. Sommers and J. Launer (eds), *Clinical Uncertainty in Primary Care: The Challenge of Collaborative Engagement*. New York: Springer, pp. 147–161.

Miller, L. (2012) Medical conversations inviting change. *Context*, 19, 16–19.

Proctor, B. (2010) Training for the supervision alliance: attitude, skills and intention. In J. Cutcliffe, J.K. Hyrkas and J. Fowler (eds), *Routledge Handbook of Clinical Supervision: Fundamental International Themes*. London: Routledge, pp. 23–34.

Whiting, J. (2007) Authors, artists and social constructionism: a case study of narrative super-vision. *American Journal of Family Therapy*, 35, 139–150.

CHAPTER NINE

Consultancy in the workplace

Key ideas in this chapter

- Professionals in health and social care often report that they are more preoccupied with issues in their work setting than they are with cases.
- Practitioners can help each other with workplace concerns, either by consulting with someone from their own team or organisation, or with colleagues from elsewhere.
- Narrative practice can be applied in work consultancy and team facilitation, using the same stance and techniques as in casework and supervision.
- Providing help of this kind for individuals or teams may be essential to enable some professionals to work effectively as clinicians, supervisors, educators or managers.

Introduction

If health and social care professionals have a pressing need to give and receive supervision on their cases, as described in the previous chapter, they also have a need to talk about the issues that arise in their teams and workplaces, and their roles there. This chapter is about such issues, and ways of helping with them by using a narrative approach. A narrative approach to consulting with colleagues about work issues is similar to the approach to supervision. The same overall concepts apply. The same techniques are effective. Helping others to create good narratives about their work also helps them to create good narratives with patients and clients. Indeed, one of the most compelling arguments for providing professional support for practitioners is that they may not have the capacity to help others to construct coherent narratives if their own stories as practitioners and team members are shot through with confusions, uncertainties or distress.

During the years that we have taught "Conversations Inviting Change," two themes have come up consistently. The first is that professionals often find the challenges of their teams and workplaces more difficult to address than the case-work itself. The second is that once they have encountered a narrative-based approach, they find it just as helpful and effective with such issues as they do with cases. Indeed, when we give practitioners the opportunity to bring narratives either about clients or about colleagues, the majority of stories they bring will often relate to dilemmas they are facing in relation to the workplace. Thus, a great deal of our activity effectively consists of mutual work consultancy. It is often through that medium that learners best acquire narrative skills. Such skills can then also be used not only to assist individual colleagues in supervision, but to help in team functioning and conflict resolution, or applied in action learning sets (Campbell and Huffington, 2008; Leonard and Marquand, 2010; Launer, 2015). Depending on circumstances, it may be possible to do this not only within one's own team or organisation, but also with colleagues from elsewhere.

A number of issues commonly emerge in work consultancy. The following sections describe a representative sample of these, with illustrative cases to demonstrate ways of addressing them through a narrative-based approach. The cases are all drawn from practitioners who attended courses and workshops in "Conversations Inviting Change" or who have applied a narrative-based approach in their work. They have been disguised in the same way as the clinical cases elsewhere.

Managing hierarchies

Not surprisingly, many of the narratives that practitioners tell concern the difficulties of managing juniors or – just as commonly – the challenges of being managed. Professionals often characterise seniors as being out of touch or autocratic, while those who actually hold senior positions may describe their subordinates as underperforming or failing to follow guidance. It is not difficult for professionals with higher status to devalue the perspectives and insights of others in less powerful positions. Equally, staff at the grass roots may not appreciate the pressures on management. Narrative-based practice can help practitioners explore the realities of others' work and build a subtler weave of shared understandings as they discover how to use each other's different perspectives.

Case example: caught in the middle

A probation officer working as a team manager described to one of our course groups how she felt caught in the middle between her own line manager and the officers on her team who were working more at the "coalface." She spoke of being under constant pressure from above to make sure her staff implemented new schedules for seeing clients, saying that she was also being encouraged to "weed out" those who were failing to do so – using disciplinary procedures where necessary. At the same time, the message from the probation officers in the community was that they were overstretched and demoralised. It was clear to her that dismissals could only make things worse. Narrative-based questioning from her course group helped her to consider how she might present the new schedules to her juniors as a potential source of job satisfaction rather than as hurdles to be jumped over. The group also helped her to plan how she could give her line manager a dispassionate story of her team's difficulties, neither understating it nor appearing to obstruct change. Interestingly, her discussion with the group led her to entertain the possibility that her line manager might himself feel under enormous pressure from the top level of management. He might even appreciate having a well-constructed narrative concerning morale in the workforce, in order to justify slowing down the pace of change.

Negotiating the roles of different professionals

When professionals talk about everyday encounters, they often tell of how these take place in a matrix of professional interactions – in the team, the organisation, or the wider system. Health and social care workers seem to be acutely aware that their job involves not just managing the interaction with the client or family. It also means managing a range of interprofessional interactions, and making sure that the combined effect of these is to produce a coherent and affirming story for the patient (Greenwood, 2016). Because of the nature of their roles, professionals can often give examples of times when they have had to sort out gaps in care. They sometimes describe these gaps in terms of perceived deficiencies in other professions, along with judgements about the way other practitioners have behaved. Narrative skills can help to address such differences and judgements, by encouraging others to gain a more appreciative stance both of themselves and their colleagues, and to find a way of telling a more nuanced story. The following case gives an example of using a narrative-based approach in this way.

Case example: an encounter between health and social services

A senior health visitor told us how a junior colleague had asked her for advice as she was concerned about two under-fives whose mother sometimes appeared to be drunk. The junior described how she had made a safeguarding referral to social services but then heard nothing for several weeks. Eventually, she received a phone call from social services inquiring about the "level of surveillance" she was currently maintaining with the family. The junior felt this was an inappropriate inquiry as surveillance was not part of her role, but also felt guilty that she had not seen the family again, since she felt she had handed them over to the social workers, and wanted to know how her colleague thought she should respond. Instead of giving her advice, her senior colleague asked her a series of questions that invited her to think about her role and responsibilities in relation to this family, and those of the social worker. In responding to these questions, the junior health visitor recognised that local social services were under considerable strain and might be unable to respond as promptly as she wished, so she should review the family in person and offer them ongoing support. She also resolved to contact the social worker to clarify that health visitors do not have any right to carry out surveillance of families, and to make sure that social services accepted the need to proceed with an appropriate child protection investigation as soon as possible.

Dealing with organisational change

Organisational change plays a large part in the narratives we hear about everyday work. Professionals bring stories about teams that have grown or shrunk in response to local and governmental pressures. Similarly, people talk of how their networks or organisations have been reconfigured multiple times, often without enough preparatory work, or opportunities for those involved to absorb what is happening or reflect on this. While a narrative-based approach may not be able to alter administrative decisions, appropriate conversations can help professionals to consider how to respond to them, and what their range of options may be, as the following example shows.

Case example: managing in a reorganised job

A youth worker asked two social workers in a training workshop in "Conversations Inviting Change" to help her to think through a work dilemma. She formerly worked in a local centre that covered a specific geographical area, and she found this very satisfying. Following a recent policy decision by area managers, however, she had now been assigned to two different centres for half the week each. The staff in one of these centres seemed to have little knowledge or understanding of her role or why she had been allocated there. As a result, she felt isolated and unsupported there. The two colleagues used a variety of open questions to allow her to talk about her frustration, and to explore the different options open to her. As a result, she decided to talk about her frustration to the area managers, and ask them to follow through their original decision with sufficient training and liaison to make it work. She recognised that this might still not have any impact, leaving her with a difficult choice for the future: to ask for a transfer, to grin and bear it, or to resign. She also used the conversation with the social workers to consider what she might need to look out for to determine if her job conditions were improving or had become unacceptable.

Improving motivation

People working in health and social care often describe working in teams or networks where everyone feels demoralised or appears to be poorly motivated. These stories may sometimes become personalised, with descriptions of colleagues who "belong to the old guard" or are seen as "incapable of change." In offering consultancy to colleagues in such circumstances, it is often necessary to explore the history, values and ethos of the workplace, in order to bring out a narrative of collaboration rather than competition and conflict.

Case example: struggling to motivate colleagues

A care home manager took the opportunity at one of our workshops to express dissatisfaction at not being able to motivate her staff to fill in incident reports for falls by elderly residents. She contrasted this with their enthusiasm for submitting forms to claim overtime or request annual leave. She had only arrived in her post fairly recently, and knew that the home had previously been poorly managed. She expressed a general sense of unhappiness at the way that self-interest seemed to dominate the behaviour of her staff. So far, she had had little contact with senior management, whom she described as "remote and focused on profits." Using only open questions, the other members of the training workshop invited her to speculate on how the historical and commercial contexts might have led to the attitudes she described. In the conversation that followed, it became clear to the care home manager that she needed to do far more groundwork, and attempt to build better relationships both with management and staff, rather than focusing at this stage on specific issues such as form-filling.

Meeting targets and bringing about quality improvement

A recurring issue in discussions between professionals is how to integrate the work of looking after specific individuals and families with the need to follow wider initiatives for delivering care, particularly in relation to measurable targets or improvements in quality. It can be tempting for practitioners to fall into opposing camps as "traditionalists" or "modernisers," and for them to see each other in negative terms as a result. A narrative-based approach can help colleagues to reframe these differences in more positive terms, and to see that effective care may depend on balancing the two perspectives, as the next case example shows.

Case example: a dentist caught in the middle

A dentist of South Asian origin, working as a sole practitioner, attended a "learning set" of local colleagues, facilitated by one of its members trained in narrative skills. The dentist explained how he had recently been elected as a representative to its executive. His constituency was largely made up of dentists from similar backgrounds to his own, also working as sole practitioners, and practising in traditional ways without much staff support. He realised that his colleagues on the executive, mostly white practitioners from larger and more sophisticated dental practices, were expecting him to pressurise his peers to accept a wide range of auditing. At the same time, his peers themselves wanted him to persuade the CCG that most patients simply wanted the kind of familiar personal service they were currently getting from their dentists. Helped by the group facilitator, the members of the learning set helped him to think about the way he could use his unusual position, with connections and allegiances to both sides, to help each recognise and harness the other's strengths.

Establishing boundaries about confidentiality

One of the most important things that health and social care professionals can offer to service users is a space to explore and create multiple stories. Clients can try out different ways of reframing their experiences with different members of the same team, or with professionals from different agencies. However, one issue raised by such multiple stories is that of confidentiality (Launer, 2005). People have a right to privacy, professional intimacy and respect for their autonomy when they discuss the same events with different practitioners. On the other hand, clients know and may even expect that there will be some exchange between professionals of the information they bring. Narrative-based work consultancy can help colleagues to balance these considerations.

Case example: a dilemma over confidentiality

A pharmacist described to a group of her colleagues how she had regular contact with a schizophrenic patient who brought in his prescriptions from a nearby GP. Sometimes she knew that the patient was not cashing in his prescriptions, or that he was coming in at long intervals that suggested he was not always taking his medication. Occasionally, the patient confessed he had told doctors an untrue story – for example, that he was attending the day hospital or seeing his psychiatric nurse, when this was not the case. Her professional relationship with the GP was good, but she was aware that she had a duty of confidentiality to her customers and did not want to get into a collusive alliance simply because the patient had a mental health issue. The colleagues used narrative inquiry to help the pharmacist clarify in her own mind what would be a legitimate reason for informing the GP. This included the need to check a change in medication, or detecting any clear evidence that the patient was putting himself or others at risk. The pharmacist also recognised it would not be legitimate to say that the patient was telling different stories to herself and others – something that she recognised anyone had the right to do if they wished.

Tolerating differences in personal values

One striking aspect of the narratives that people tell about their work in health and social care is the closeness in their minds between the professional and the personal. In the safe context of a learning group, individuals may talk both about the work itself and about the personal connections and beliefs that help them to make sense of it. For example, professionals who were once refugees or migrants speak of how they apply their own experiences of displacement to working with a later influx of refugees from different places. Practitioners with strong religious beliefs have disclosed how much their community ties and commitment inform their work. Lesbian, gay, bisexual or transgender practitioners have explained how marginalisation has sharpened their understanding of many of their clients. People who are parents often refer to the importance of their own experience of raising children and how they apply this experience in their work. Those who have nursed sick or dying parents, who have been through serious illnesses, or who have been subject to political or social discrimination, have reflected on the way this has changed their own attitudes or practice.

While respecting sensitivities and allowing people to remain silent, narrative practitioners can offer people permission to make connections between their professional and personal lives. This opens the possibility of a seamless story that makes sense of what people do in health and social care, and why they do it.

Case example: scroungers or deserving poor?

A discussion in a team of paramedics on a workshop in "Conversations Inviting Change" concerned emergency calls from particular kinds of patients who were perceived to be "feeble." Some people in the team took exception to this description, saying that it was important to try to understand why certain patients seemed to call ambulances for apparently trivial reasons. They argued that one could never know exactly what patients' subjective suffering might be. Some of them spoke of personal experiences in their families or origin that led them to take a more "liberal" view of why people used public services, and why they were inclined to take every request at face value. When the workshop facilitator asked if there were any other views in the room, two paramedics in the team with more "conservative" beliefs said that they believed that everyone had responsibilities to society as well as rights. What motivated them in their own work, they said, was a commitment to fairness and justice, but they expected this from their patients as well as themselves. Some of them mentioned examples of how they had overcome adversity by their own efforts and felt it was reasonable to ask others to be less dependent too. The group had never discussed these differences in experiences and attitudes before, other than in brief exchanges of banter. They then talked about whether both points of view could be held harmoniously within the same team, and came to the conclusion that it was fine to do so.

Facilitating better teamwork

Many teams in health and social care work in highly pressurised conditions, where the decisions they make are critical to others' lives and may literally be a matter of life and death. In these circumstances, personal and professional relationships can come under strain, and interactions become tense or adversarial. If used sensitively and with skill, a non-judgemental, narrative-based approach can help team members gain an understanding of how such dynamics arise, and learn to manage these in ways that can improve the work ethos and contribute to improved care.

Case example: changing the culture on an intensive care unit

Two trainers with experience of applying a narrative approach were asked to work with a multidisciplinary group of staff on an intensive care unit. A survey of staff had shown evidence of an "abrasive" culture, with younger members feeling silenced and sometimes intimidated. The trainers encouraged the exchange of a variety of different attitudes to the work environment, which was clearly pressurised and emotionally demanding. The more assertive senior members spoke about their desire for rigorous standards when dealing with patients' life-threatening conditions, and how they wished to develop robustness in their less experienced colleagues so they could learn to cope with this. The younger and less confident team members also had the opportunity to speak about occasions when they had wanted to ask questions to help with their own learning, or to draw attention to concerns about case management, but had met with dismissive responses and "just ordered around." Over the course of several meetings, the facilitators helped the team to find common ground in their wish for the unit to be known for its clinical excellence. They also helped the team establish that this required a variety of interactional styles at different times, including a clear hierarchy and direct orders at moments that were medically critical, but more ability to accept dialogue and challenge at other times, especially during case presentations and handover between shifts. A staff survey following the work with the team showed a significant improvement in work satisfaction among both senior and younger members. Several respondents also commented that they felt that patient care was better as a result of more openness to hearing different opinions in case discussions.

Suggested exercises

1 When a colleague next tells you about a work difficulty, ask if you can offer support through a narrative approach and questioning rather than through sympathy and advice.
2 Next time a dilemma at work arises, consider how you might approach it from a different perspective. For example, ask a colleague if you can have a confidential discussion to develop your thinking about it. Or use a group setting away from your workplace to ask for some independent consideration of the dilemma.
3 If there are professionals in your network who do consultancy work of any kind, consider asking if they have availability to act as a resource to help people in the workplace think about concerns that are wider than clinical ones.

References

Campbell, D. and Huffington, C. (eds) (2008) *Organisations Connected: A Handbook of Systemic Consultation*. London: Karnac.

Greenwood, J. (2016) Influencing systems. In L. Smith (ed.), *Clinical Practice at the Edge of Care: Developments in Working with At-Risk Children and Their Families*. London: Palgrave Macmillan, pp. 29–47.

Launer, J. (2005) Introduction. In J. Launer, S. Blake and D. Daws (eds), *Reflecting on Reality: Psychotherapists at Work in Primary Care*. London: Karnac, pp. 1–17.

Launer, J. (2015) Concentric conversations. *Postgraduate Medical Journal*, 91, 177–178.

Leonard, H.S. and Marquand, M.J. (2010) The evidence for the effectiveness of action learning. *Action Learning: Research and Practice*, 7(2), 121–136.

CHAPTER TEN

Training

Key ideas in this chapter

- We teach "Conversations Inviting Change" using a mixture of presentations, demonstration interviews, intensive coaching in small groups, and large group work.
- The main emphasis is on the small group work, where people bring real, live issues for discussion. We use role play only sparingly.
- In the small group work, course participants take it in turns to bring a problem, act as interviewer, or be observers. We take regular pauses in the conversation to reflect on its progress and effectiveness.
- In working with larger groups, we sometimes make use of so-called "reflecting teams," where a small subgroup of participants offer comments from time to time on the progress of a supervision conversation taking place in a "fishbowl."
- There is independent evidence to show that training in "Conversations Inviting Change" can help participants make significant progress in their work as supervisors.

Introduction

As an approach to professional work, "Conversations Inviting Change" comes alive only in conversations between professionals and their clients, or between professionals themselves. This chapter gives an account of how we teach the approach, mainly by helping practitioners to learn and apply it through supervising each other while being observed and coaching. The mainstay of "Conversations Inviting Change" consists of our interactive courses. While these cannot be captured fully by any written account, conversely it is impossible to grasp the approach to any significant extent without reading about how we run our live trainings and why we do it a particular way.

Core training

Our core training takes place over three days (London Deanery, 2012). Rather than running it on consecutive days, we generally do so with an interval or one or two weeks between each of the training days. This gives participants time to digest the ideas, practise them, do the required reading, and bring their experiences and questions to the next training day. We also run one-day workshops and even occasionally half-day tasters. However, from experience, we have come to believe that it takes a minimum of three days' training spread over a few weeks for people to grasp the attitude we are trying to impart, as well as some of the skills. One of the reasons for this is that participants often arrive with a prior conviction that they are already well versed in approaches to interactional skills that they believe to be "person-centred," and it takes time for them to understand quite how radical a shift we are attempting to bring about in their ability to notice the subtleties by which people communicate their realities, and in their capacity to respond to these without unexamined assumptions or the unconscious application of their professional power and authority.

Whatever the length of training, we try to keep a very low ratio between trainers and participants, ideally with one trainer for every four participants. This means that a great deal of the work can be done by close coaching in small groups. Where economics or logistics do not allow this, a smaller number of trainers may need to move between small groups, but as a result they will not be able to monitor everything that goes on in each group or provide input exactly when it is needed. Hence, for a group of 16 people, we will generally try to deploy a training team of four accredited "CIC" trainers. One of them, usually one of the more experienced trainers, acts as a lead to oversee the planning for the course.

Although we sometimes work with a group of course participants where everyone knows each other (for example, a group of paramedic educators in one city), in general this is not the case. Instead, the intake is more likely to consist of people from different organisations and backgrounds who have signed up for the course individually. A typical course group might consist, for example, of one or two psychiatrists or psychologists, a couple of social workers, three or four GPs, a counsellor or hospice worker, some hospital consultants from a variety of specialties, and a health service manager. Many participants are likely to have teaching roles in their own work settings, as well as being interested in applying the approach in their clinical work. All have come voluntarily, many because of recommendations from colleagues. Although some of the courses are accredited with points that may count towards someone's annual requirement for continuing professional development, participants always have options, and we are keen to ensure that no one ever comes compulsorily.

We alert participants in advance to the fact that the course is experiential, and ask them to bring narratives from their own work experience, using the instructions that appear in Box 10.1.

Box 10.1   Preparation for supervision skills training

As part of training, we will be using real-life scenarios (not role play) for most of the day. In order to do this, we need you to provide the material. This helps to make the course relevant and also provides you with an opportunity to get help with situations that are not yet resolved in your own workplace. Please take a few minutes to think about the question below and jot down your ideas about what you might discuss. We will use the real-life scenarios in the demonstration of supervision or in the small group work. The question we want you to answer is as follows:

What current dilemmas do I have that I would benefit from "working through" with a supportive colleague? This can be in relation to your work as a practitioner, a teacher in your discipline, a team member or a manager. The scenario needs to be:

- *current* (not already solved or in the past);
- *real* (not hypothetical or imaginary);
- *your own* (not someone else's problem);
- *individual* (dealing with a specific person or team, not a generic issue); and
- *hot* (causing you concern, but it also needs to be suitable for sharing in confidence with the group).

These instructions have been framed as tightly as we can. In spite of this, some participants may still arrive expecting to discuss rather vague topics such as "How can I motivate my trainees?" or "How can my department get better funding?" This may be because extended, case-based discussion is now so unusual for some practitioners that it is hard for them even to recognise what will be required of them on an experiential course such as this.

Direct teaching

Following a brief explanation of some ground rules (confidentiality, not taking phone calls, and so on), we often open a course with a "bonding" exercise, such as asking everyone to say something about a geographical place that means a great deal to them, and why this is the case. While we plan for most of each course to be interactional, we have found that participants expect at least a brief introduction to the theoretical principles and benefits of the approach, in order to understand what they have subscribed to. One of the team members therefore always gives a talk at the outset for perhaps 20 minutes, providing some theoretical background and other essential information about the course. During this, we explain that we use mutual peer supervision as our principal way of helping people learn the approach – in the belief that working in real time with genuine, live narratives of people's work experiences is the most effective way of learning it, and makes it easier to extrapolate it to other settings, including clinical ones.

We then explain how supervision, like clinical work, always has two aspects to it: one that involves deep listening and matching responses, and another that involves performing a professional task that may need to include instructional teaching. In the initial presentation, we address the principles of narrative-based supervision, but we do so without using technical words we may want to introduce later on, such as hypothesising. We restrict ourselves instead to introducing "the seven C's," using the summary that appears earlier in this book in Box 1.1.

During the rest of the course, we will carry out a small amount of additional direct teaching and ask people to do some reading – including an "Introduction to theory." However, the main message we hope to demonstrate and to model during the course is that the approach is entirely focused on responsiveness and precision in human interaction, and hence can only be learned through that modality as well. One of the things we demonstrate consistently during the course is that the teaching team will be in constant dialogue with each other about how things are progressing, and how and when to do different activities. We have many of these exchanges transparently in front of the whole course group – even to the extent of expressing different points of view among ourselves. We also meet privately in the breaks, at lunchtime and at the end of the day, to provide each other as a team with mutual support and supervision. We use this time, for example, to think how to address differences in skill levels between different course participants, or how to help a course member who is having difficulty integrating with the group, or has brought dilemmas from their workplace that seem particularly complex or distressing.

Demonstrating the approach

As part of the direct teaching on the first morning of any course, we give a demonstration of supervision using "Conversations Inviting Change." We ask for a member of the participants' group to volunteer to have a conversation with one of the members of the teaching team, with everyone else on the course observing this in the manner of a "fishbowl." Usually, several course participants will volunteer to bring a narrative that they have thought about as a result of the instructions that were given before the course, so we ask each of them to give a summary of their "case" in two or three sentences. We then try to choose the one that we believe may be best for demonstration purposes. This choice may be governed by purely practical factors such as a clear voice and good English, but we also take into account other considerations – for example, not choosing the most senior or confident person present, or a problem that sounds as if it might be amenable to a purely technical solution, or one that may have serious legal implications. The reason for being selective in this way is so we can demonstrate how helpful the approach is for drawing out the complexity of everyday work and addressing this with as few distractions as possible in the initial stage of learning.

This demonstration usually takes around 20 minutes. Afterwards, we invite course participants to comment on what they have observed. Many participants, out of sheer habit, go straight into problem-solving mode, or at the very least focus immediately on specific details in the narrative itself, or start offering advice to the volunteer about what they should do. We try to steer people away from this, and encourage them to comment instead on what has taken place in the interaction itself. What we are trying to do here is to alert people to the way meaning and narrative develop through the conversational interchange between people, so that they can then begin to reorient themselves to this perspective while they acquire skills on the rest of the course.

Small supervision groups

Most of the time on any course is spent in practising "Conversations Inviting Change" in small supervision groups of four or five people. This is the medium through which learners will acquire and apply the key ideas and skills of the approach. The members of each small group take it in turns to adopt the roles of: (a) the "narrator" (who brings an account of a challenge they are facing in the workplace); (b) the "supervisor" or "interviewer" (who takes on the task of engaging in a one-to-one conversation with the narrator); and (c) the "observer" (or observers). In each episode of supervision, which may take 20 or 30 minutes, the narrator will have an opportunity to expand on their specific difficulty, receive supervision on it, and consider ways forward. In accordance with the instructions in Box 10.1, the narrator can choose whether to bring a scenario based on their work as a practitioner, a teacher, a team member or a manager. Conversely, the supervisor will be able to practise the techniques that they are here to learn, and the observer(s) can watch the process at work.

Each of the small supervision groups on a course is also assigned a member of the teaching team who acts as a coach. It is the coach's role to make sure the group works effectively and safely, and progresses in its learning. The coaching role includes, among other things, checking that the narratives that are brought are suitable ones, not too vague or general, and that every member of the small group in turn has a chance to take on the position of narrator, supervisor and observer. It also includes ensuring care and safety so that the emerging conversation does not delve into the realm of amateur therapy, and ensuring that narrators have permission to stop the conversation if they choose. The coach may need to reiterate – often more than once – that the members of the group are *not* being asked to role-play. Quite the contrary, this is what has been described as "real play," where the stories being brought by narrators are genuine, current and live ones, and everyone is precisely whom they appear to be: experienced professionals from different backgrounds, here in the moment, and being themselves.

A key part of the coach's role is also to "freeze" the conversation from time to time, to invite the supervisor to comment on their own performance (for example, how well they are managing to ask open and creative questions), and to think about alternative ways of inquiring into the narrative. So far as possible during these intervals, coaches will try to use exactly the same questioning approach in the way they converse with learners that they hope the learners will increasingly adopt with each other and, in due course, with their colleagues, patients and clients. Over time, the coach who works with any small group will also gradually introduce a variety of different techniques to help the group advance. This will include, for example, taking pauses in the conversation not only for the supervisor to comment on their performance, but to invite the observer(s) to say what they are curious about, and to contribute hypotheses or possible questions.

For the initial rounds of the small group work, we give the "supervisor" the following instructions. Sometimes we call these the "narrative default position" or the "golden rules":

- Only ask questions – and try to keep these simple and short.
- Make sure that each question links directly with something the narrator has already said.
- Withhold any suggestions, advice or interpretations, or test these out tentatively by questioning; offer them directly only at the end of the conversation, and only if the supervisor requests this.

We do not mean to imply that these are the *only* ways to conduct a professional encounter, a piece of supervision, or even a narrative-based conversation. Quite the contrary, we will encourage people as each course progresses to integrate other approaches that they have been using professionally, sometimes for many years, so that the way they use "Conversations Inviting Change" for themselves will be more natural, personal and spontaneous. At the same time, we have always found that it is essential for people to stick to these "golden rules" in the early stages of their learning. This helps them to notice their own habitual ways of responding in conversations, and to observe how this may inhibit narrative progression rather than enabling it. They also discover, nearly always to their own considerable surprise, how difficult it is to follow a conversational discipline that seems as apparently easy as the one that these three rules represent. It is generally only when they have gone through this process that they are ready to experiment and improvise with ways of owning "Conversations Inviting Change" that is not just an unintentional way of reverting to what may be quite controlling or paternalistic ways of interacting.

A small group at work

This section gives an extended description of a typical small group at work. It conveys what actually happens in narrative-based supervision. Although detailed, it is worth reading for anyone who wants to gain an impression of what the live work is like. Members of our teaching group who have read it have commented that it captures the essence of our approach more than the abstract descriptions of it (the account is adapted with permission from Launer, 2013).

The group in this description (a fictionalised one, distilled from many real ones) consists of a team member called Salima, a GP by background who is acting as a coach, and three group participants: Barry, Wesley and Kate. Kate is a family planning nurse and she offers to bring a clinical case that is bothering her – a young woman she has seen the previous day. Barry, a senior social worker, offers to supervise her on this. Salima as coach helps them to rearrange the seating. Barry and Kate face each other as supervisor and narrator. Wesley, a surgeon, sits alongside Barry as an observer, and Salima sits a very small distance away from the group, but where she can see all three of them clearly.

Barry begins his inquiry by posing some questions he has noted from the demonstration supervision that he observed earlier that morning:

"What do I need to know about you or your team, to make sense of what you're going to tell me?"

"Which other professionals are involved in this case?"

[Comment: People are often struck by the emphasis we place on understanding contexts before going for content, and by the way we encourage carefully graded questions of the kind Barry has asked here. Such questions help to build trust, especially between colleagues who may not know each other. They establish information that might otherwise turn out to be essential later – but only when the supervisor has already advanced too far on the basis of incorrect assumptions.

They also encourage the narrator to start conceptualising the problem from an interactional point of view.]

Having found out about the work setting, Barry next asks Kate to tell him about her client. She tells him about a 16-year-old girl called Cherie whom she has seen a number of times. Cherie has already had multiple sexual partners, is casual about contraception, and is possibly a substance abuser, although she denies this. As it happens, Kate also knows and sees Cherie's mother, who is HIV-positive and on a methadone programme. Cherie and her mother seem to have a lot of secrets from each other, which Kate feels is unhealthy.

Kate now elaborates on the mother's history, going into detail. Barry nods encouragingly, frequently says "Mmm" and looks highly engaged, but he does not pose any further questions. Salima, the coach, requests the group's permission to "freeze-frame" the conversation, and asks Barry what is going through his mind:

Barry: I'm feeling a bit overwhelmed. I thought my opening questions were good but now I'm not sure if I should interrupt. She said she wanted to talk about Cherie but now she's only talking about the mother.

Salima: What do you think Kate wants from this conversation?

Barry: To be honest, at this moment I haven't a clue!

[Comment: Barry is a "good listener." However, Kate needs more than "just listening." If all that Barry does is to listen without asking some questions to help her focus her thoughts, he may be infected by Kate's own apparent sense of being overwhelmed, without offering her any chance of developing a different narrative. Salima's intervention was effectively a teaching point to draw his attention to this process.]

Barry turns back to Kate and asks her why she brought the case to supervision and what she wants to get out of it. Kate, who has heard Salima's exchange with Barry, is clearly relieved by the question. She says there are two related things that are really bothering her about the case. First, Cherie is refusing to give a blood sample for HIV and drug testing, even though the results would make a big difference to the kind of help Kate could offer. Second, Kate would like to enlist the mother's help in persuading her to do so, but doesn't know if it's possible to do this without the risk of breaking confidences on both sides.

The conversation progresses. Barry does well in exploring these dilemmas. Some of his questions seem to imitate types of question that were asked in the demonstration earlier, but miss the mark as far as Kate concerned. Others are spot on, including an inquiry about how she has managed in similar sets of circumstances in the past. After a while, Salima pauses the conversation again to ask Barry how he thinks he is doing. He reflects that the supervision seems to be moving forward.

Salima agrees and congratulates him on some particularly telling questions. She also says she would now like to bring the observer into the conversation. She asks Wesley "What are you noticing? Have you had any thoughts about other questions that Barry might ask Kate?"

Wesley is clearly pleased to have been brought into the exercise. He was looking a bit bored (which is one of the reasons Salima intervened as she did), and now offers a list of things he thinks Kate should and should not do. He talks about informed consent in relation to the blood tests, rules of confidentiality in relation to 16-year-olds and their parents, and how careful you have to be to avoid complaints these days. Salima asks him "Could you turn any of those points into a question for Barry to ask?" Wesley looks puzzled and says "No, I think Barry is doing just fine. But Kate needs to be jolly careful with these two women. I got into hot water in a case just like this."

[Comment: Some course participants apparently cannot observe the *process* of a conversation as well as the content, and they cannot stop themselves from giving advice. When this happens, the main responsibility of the coach is to keep everyone focused on the main tasks, namely to make sure the narrator had appropriate help with her dilemmas, and that the supervisor learns some new skills. When this particular observer gets his chance to act as supervisor in the afternoon, the coach may need to intervene more often and be more directive with him. If a course member is still not "getting it" on the second day, the team will discuss how to address this at a debriefing during a break.]

Salima turns back to Barry and recommends the standard tactic used at this point in narrative-based supervision. Rather than choosing the next question himself, he might just ask Kate what is going through her mind at the moment, or if there is anything she has heard in the group conversation that has given her some new ideas.

To the surprise of both Salima and Barry, Kate says that she has found some of Wesley's ideas helpful. They have made her realise that she had overcommitted herself in her own mind to a campaign of persuasion in relation to both Cherie and her mother: persuading Cherie to have blood tests, persuading them to talk to each other more, persuading the mother to persuade the daughter, and so on. "Maybe I should chill out and let Cherie make her own choices. I could try to build up trust with her like I did with her mum. Anyway, I need to read up more on confidentiality and when you can breach it. I take risks sometimes and I know I shouldn't."

Barry is curious about Kate's response. Picking up on her phrases, he asks her what "chilling out" with Cherie would involve, and how Kate would know when she has "built up trust." Following her responses to these questions, he asks her where she thinks she might find up-to-date information about confidentiality and when to breach it. "Perhaps I can ask Wesley over lunch," she replies, and all four of them laugh.

Salima, sensing a good moment to finish, suggests that Barry should ask Kate to review what she has got out of the conversation. She says she feels far more relaxed about the situation, and is actually now beginning to think of personal reasons why she was so exercised by it in the first place. Barry blushes and says "Did I miss something important?" Kate replies "No, I don't want to talk about it here – it's about my own daughter and a problem she's been having. I don't want to go into it, but it was really helpful to make the link. I wouldn't have thought of it without your questions."

Salima asks Wesley to offer his comments. He says he is pleased his counsel was helpful, and disarms everyone by apologising for getting "carried away" earlier, because of his own previous experience of a complaint. Finally, Barry reviews his own performance. In retrospect, he says he thinks the context-setting questions at the beginning were probably unnecessary. He also explains he has learned a lot from Wesley's comments: you can deprive people by not giving advice when they actually want it, and sometimes "being carried away" spontaneously may be more effective than sticking to the rules. He also confesses that he might have "gone for the jugular" with his own supervisees in social work, asking them straight away who the girl or her mother reminded them of in their own families, and possibly making it more difficult for them to reflect on this as a result.

[Comment: This vignette demonstrates the potential of narrative-based supervision to generate unexpected learning. It also shows how hard it is to pin down what is "right" and "wrong" in supervision. There are no simple rules about how to integrate a purely narrative approach with more conventional ones such as giving advice or making direct personal inquiries. What small group work such as this allows people to discover is how complex a task this can be, and how to adapt to each person and dilemma from moment to moment.]

Large group work and reflecting teams

In addition to the small group work, our courses also include supervision in larger groups. We do this in order to show that large group discussions can be more effective if carried out using a narrative-based approach, and conducted in a more structured manner than is often the case. They can also be even better than small groups in drawing people's attention to the multiple perspectives than can always be taken on any individual's dilemma, and how helpful it can be to stimulate dialogue about these. Our basic application of this method involves having a narrator and supervisor sitting in front of the whole course group, facing each other. In the same way as happens with small group work, the narrator will give an account of the issue or dilemma that they want to talk about, and the task of the supervisor is to question them about it in a way that will allow new elements of the narrative to emerge. A coach sits next to the supervisor, making the same kinds of interventions that they would make in small group work. Similarly, the coach will ask the narrator and supervisor to take pauses in the conversation from time to time, so that the supervisor can reflect on what is happening and consider how to take the conversation forward.

The significant difference from small group work is that, as well as these three individuals, a team of five or six observers (from among the whole course group) will be sitting close to the supervisor and coach, watching and listening to the interview, and prepared to act as a "reflecting team" when requested (Andersen, 1987; Launer, 2016). When there is a pause in the conversation, the supervisor and coach have the opportunity not only to talk to each other, but also to engage the reflecting team in conversation, seek their hypotheses about the matter under discussion, or suggestions concerning further questions that might take the conversation forward. The members of the reflecting team may then hold a conversation just among themselves that the narrator and supervisor can listen in to passively. Alternatively, the supervisor and narrator may want to join in their conversation. Generally speaking, narrators never take part in this discussion. This allows them to take a break from being the central focus of the supervision, and also to listen in to the multiple views or ideas that members of the reflecting team are generating. Occasionally, a narrator makes a straightforward request for the team to give advice, but the general rule with reflecting teams is the same as it is with small groups, namely to withhold advice to the end.

After each pause to hear a reflecting team discussion, the supervisor will, as a routine, ask the narrator "Is there anything you've heard from the reflecting team that you'd like to respond to?" and "Have you had any other new thoughts of your own?" The rationale for this is that the narrator may well have picked up different ideas from the team discussion than the ones the supervisor considered most significant, or may have gone off on their own train of thought and reached an entirely different place in relation to the dilemma under discussion.

Above all, this permits the narrator to keep control of their own emerging story, rather than to feel that the supervisor and the reflecting team are dominating or colonising it.

When the whole supervision is finished, the coach will generally ask everyone in turn – the supervisor, the narrator, the reflecting team and then the wider course group – what they have each learned from their own perspective. We also ask everyone not to discuss the case further once the supervision discussion is finished. Our purpose in making this request is to prevent people from reverting to familiar forms of advice-giving, or intruding on people with their own strong views when they may need reflective time to process the thinking they have done during the supervision itself. It also signifies a boundary in terms of confidentiality.

With very large course groups, we may break the participants up so we can conduct two or more reflecting team exercises of this kind in different rooms. Alternatively, we might ask some participants to observe the whole exercise – including the reflecting team – through a video link. When it is finished, they will then have an opportunity to return to talk about their observations of the process that took place while the supervisor, narrator and reflecting team were at work.

In a limited set of circumstances, we do introduce role-play exercises. For example, in a group where a number of members report struggling with an under-performing junior, we might invite one of them to act the part of the junior in question, while other members of the group take it in turns to experiment with different ways of engaging with them conversationally, and course members are invited to comment on what seems to be most effective. However, we find improvisatory work of this kind needs to be quite carefully choreographed, in order to prevent it degenerating into comedy or confrontation, or lacking in verisimilitude.

In another approach to practising "Conversations Inviting Change," we also engage in an exercise we call "speed supervision." Here, members of the course group pair off and take it in turns to supervise each other, for exactly five minutes each, on a minor everyday dilemma (e.g. "I don't know where to go on my next holiday" or "I can't decide whether to get a dog"). This exercise is effective as an energiser and also an opportunity for people to discover how the techniques might be applied in a very short space of time. A selection of further exercises appears in the Appendix.

Training the trainers

Because of the demand for training in "Conversations Inviting Change," we have periodically run part-time courses for trainers in the method, lasting between six months and a year. We generally require candidates to have attended a three-day course previously, and to have performed well on this, as well as having opportunities in their own work to apply and transmit the approach. On the "Training the Trainers" courses, we use an extended range of reading and theoretical presentations (many of these by participants), but the core of the training remains intensive small group work – with one of the learners this time taking on the role of coach, while an experienced tutor observes them and offers feedback. People attending the courses also practise their skills by acting as team members on our one-day workshops and three-day courses, and by organising teaching in their own work contexts. They have to complete a total of at least 60 hours of teaching and keep a reflective diary of this work. This contributes to their assessment, along with a video recording of a piece of one-to-one supervision they have carried out.

Evidence from training

In the field of health and social care education, it is notoriously difficult to track the effects of complex interventions, especially those that are aimed to bring about attitudinal changes. One obvious reason for this difficulty is that practitioners are exposed to such multifactorial influences – in their work and management support as well as their continuing professional development – that it is effectively impossible in many cases to exclude these variables when trying to determine which particular component of their education may have had positive effects. When teaching an approach such as "Conversations Inviting Change," an additional challenge is that this has taken place in many different organisational contexts, where the cultures and system-wide attitudes may be entirely different, and the effects of a training in one place not necessarily reproducible in another.

Having said that, there are a number of pointers to the effectiveness of our approach, most especially our success in bringing a radical view of conversations in health and social care into some mainstream institutions, including hospital and mental health trusts in the United Kingdom, as well as university departments and medical schools in many places around the world. This has exposed people within a wide range of professions to narrative ideas and skills in a way that they would be very unlikely to encounter elsewhere in their professional development. There has also been local dissemination of the approach in a number of countries, including in Scandinavia. Wider evidence comes from other, similar narrative-based approaches elsewhere. For example, in Denmark, Davidsen and Reventlow (2011, p. 966) found that:

> Doctors who took a narrative approach became more deeply involved with the patient and exhibited a greater engagement. They stressed that the narrative was the pathway to emotional engagement and empathy with the patient, and participation in co-construction of the story was considered an empathic approach.

In narrative medicine worldwide, an increasing number of studies have demonstrated the effectiveness of training medical students and clinicians in written reflections on their work, including a positive impact on doctor–patient relationships, team effectiveness, cultural understanding and affiliation with peers (Charon et al., 2016).

Our own three-day course has undergone an independent evaluation (Bullock et al., 2011) using audio and video recordings of their performance during the duration of the course. They also asked a number of participants to keep audio diaries describing their use of learned skills between course sessions. They examined all the data, focusing on three levels of learning according to a standard model of educational research:

1 reaction or satisfaction with the programme;
2 demonstration of learning; and
3 extent to which new learning is applied to practice.

The most salient findings included the following:

- Participants gave a clear endorsement of the core activity of the course: the opportunity to practise supervision in small groups. Although they found practising the new questioning techniques in these groups challenging, they valued the high-quality feedback that was generally provided by the trainers.
- Modelling of the "seven C's" by trainers was the most effective way of conveying a narrative stance. Course participants were able to apply this model even when their questioning did not necessarily "fit the rules." As a result, both trainers and participants were sometimes able to produce positive outcomes in supervision even when being didactic, so long as their overall stance was facilitative. Conversely, it was possible for some people to sometimes "talk the talk" but with negative outcomes because significant elements of the "seven C's" were lacking.
- There was variability among trainers, in participants' views of "non-core" activities such as role play, and in how well strong emotion was handled in the groups. Out of six participants studied in depth, five considered they had made progress in their own development, although analysis of their supervision performance showed this was not all equal. For example, one participant "seemed to have embodied this way of being, demonstrating an impact on himself as a person," while another "appeared to employ the techniques as a way of bringing the interactant around to a prescribed conclusion rather than enabling them to explore fully the situation for themselves."

These findings are consistent with our own experience as trainers. They fit well with the vignette of small group work earlier in this chapter, where the considered questions at the beginning of the supervision turned out to be less effective than the suggestions of someone who was apparently "breaking the rules." The report highlights that the overall tolerance of the narrative stance gives scope for even discordant interventions to bring about a positive difference, in circumstances where a purely mechanical application of narrative techniques alone would be ineffective. This matches our belief that "Conversations Inviting Change" represents a vision, not a toolbox. If any conversation takes us in a new direction, we try our best to follow it. We want this to hold true for the overall approach just as much as it does for the individual elements from which it is constituted. In the last resort, narrative-based practice can only remain true to itself if it remains as flexible and responsive as the conversations it seeks to enable.

References

Andersen, T. (1987) Dialogue and meta-dialogue in clinical work. *Family Process*, 26, 415–428.

Bullock, A., Monrouxe, L. and Atwell, C. (2011) *Evaluation of the London Deanery Training Course "Supervision Skills for Clinical Teachers" (Working Paper 141)*. Cardiff: University of Cardiff School of Social Sciences.

Charon, R., Hermann, N. and Devlin, M.J. (2016) Close reading and creative writing: teaching attention, representation and affiliation. *Academic Medicine*, 91, 345–350.

Davidsen, A.S. and Reventlow, S. (2011) Narratives about patients with psychological problems illustrate different professional roles among general practitioners. *Journal of Health Psychology*, 16, 959–968.

Launer, J. (2013) Training for narrative-based supervision: conversations inviting change. In L.S. Sommers and J. Launer (eds), *Clinical Uncertainty in Primary Care: The Challenge of Collaborative Engagement*. New York: Springer, pp. 163–176.

Launer, J. (2016) Clinical case discussion: using a reflecting team, *Postgraduate Medical Journal*, 92, 245–246.

London Deanery (2012) *Supervision Skills for Clinical Teachers: A World Class Teaching Initiative*. Available at: www.faculty.londondeanery.ac.uk/supervision-skills-for-clinical-teachers [accessed 17 May 2017].

Appendix
Some teaching exercises

The majority of our exercises on courses are based on using small supervision groups and reflecting teams, as described in Chapter 10. However, for certain occasions, including the development of some more complex skills such as working with genograms, dealing with mental health problems or interviewing couples, we use some more prescriptive exercises. We have found the following exercises particularly useful.

Active or "deep" listening

This exercise (adapted from Miller and Halpern, 2012) helps people to notice and develop habits that indicate attentiveness and emotional availability to clients:

- Course participants divide into pairs. One person in each pair is the narrator; the other is the listener.
- The narrators are invited to tell their listeners about something they have recently enjoyed or feel positive about, and that they are happy to share.
- The listeners are asked to listen in "active" or "deep" mode for 60 seconds, at which point the course facilitator will ring a bell.
- The listeners then have to change to "distraction" mode by breaking eye contact and using non-verbal behaviour to indicate that they are not listening (e.g. answering their phones, rummaging in their bags, etc.).
- After a further 60 seconds, the listeners are asked to resume "active" listening for 60 seconds.
- The pairs then swap roles and repeat the two-stage exercise.
- The pairs each feed back to the large group their observations from the position of the listener, and then go on to relate this to their consultations or professional conversations.

Normative and narrative interviewing

This exercise gives people a chance to explore the possibilities and limits of taking a narrative-based approach:

- We divide the course group into threes or fours: each small group then chooses a presenter, an interviewer and one or two observers.
- We ask each presenter to think of one particular client who has an unconventional view of their own situation (in terms of its nature, its cause or the intervention needed). The presenter in each small group then has a chance to describe that person briefly.
- We then ask the presenters to "turn themselves into the client" and take on that person's role for a consultation.
- We ask the interviewers to run the consultation twice over, allowing 10 to 15 minutes each time. The first time, we suggest that interviewers should hold on to their normal consulting style. While being reasonably tolerant of the person's unorthodox beliefs, they should continue to act on the basis that their own view of the complaint is "normative" and has absolute authority. Within the limits of normal courtesy, they should try to persuade the client of the "reality" of their situation and the reasons for recommending the intervention needed.
- For the second performance of the encounter, however, we ask interviewers to act as if they are anthropologists. We invite them to try to enter the clients' conceptual worlds without any prejudice or assumptions about what is and is not an acceptable description of reality.

The following issues usually emerge from this exercise:

1   It is very difficult to stay neutral. Even the most accomplished practitioners are surprised how hard it is to sustain a genuinely inquisitive and uncritical stance, especially when faced with beliefs or behaviour that appear to fly in the face of conventional professional wisdom. For most practitioners, knowledge of what is "true" or "right" is so deeply ingrained that they will constantly display their professional mindset, in spite of their very best efforts.

2   Clients are uncomfortable with total neutrality. One common finding in this exercise is that the "clients" find it impossible to *allow* their interviewers to remain neutral. Their own expectations of professionals are so inflexible that they anticipate that their views will be opposed, and therefore exert pressure on their interviewers to take an oppositional stance. When the interviewers do succeed in expressing permissiveness towards their beliefs, the "clients" may become quite disconcerted. This demonstrates how people sometimes need

professionals to remain within their expected social roles rather than try to "get out of the frame" through an excess of empathy.

3 Absolute neutrality causes dilemmas. Interviewers who genuinely try to demonstrate neutrality in this exercise can encounter some quite acute dilemmas. For example, they may find themselves becoming drawn into a collusive agreement with ideas that are dangerous or delusional (for example, if their client says "insulin won't help my diabetes, it will only poison me"). They may also have to grapple with the consequences of listening to a highly partisan view of the world without opposing it. Direct confrontation of such views will almost certainly fail. On the other hand, total permissiveness towards the client will completely paralyse the conversation. This experience compels the group to examine the kind of difficulty that may arise in real life with service users whose views are at variance with the professional. What the exercise invites people to discover, therefore, is how to show respectful curiosity, while still remaining able to describe – but not insist on – a professional perspective.

Learning to take genograms

We sometimes ask course groups to spend a session working in pairs on their own genograms. In health and social care consultations, the focus of a genogram is usually an attempt to gain a wider understanding of a problem. Working with colleagues, the focus is less clear, so we sometimes offer these suggestions:

- "Focus on how first names are assigned in the family, and what they mean." Most families pay careful attention to the naming of new members, and the choices made by the various generations or branches of a family can yield important meaning (e.g. the transition from religious to secular names, or a tradition of passing down the names of honoured forebears).
- "Focus on any differences of ethnicity, religion, or social class within the family, and what these differences mean." In the most seemingly homogenous families, small nuances of social or religious difference can take on enormous importance. In reality, most of the families described by any group of professionals in inner London in the early twenty-first century will reveal an astonishingly rich diversity of origins and identities.
- "Focus on trying to understand what influences within the family might have led your interviewee to choose their particular career." Practitioners may come from families with strong traditions of professional caring, but they may also come from families where illness and suffering has figured importantly, or where medical and nursing training has signified particular virtues or kinds of social achievement.

Issues that we encounter when doing this exercise include the following:

1 Nearly everyone reports finding that having their genogram elicited is a moving experience, making connections they had never previously considered, and gaining new understanding of how the past has influenced the present. Some people have been inspired by doing this to go on to do some interviews within their own families, either for historical or for personal and reparative reasons.
2 It is important for people who take each other's genograms to know they do not have to disclose any information they do not want to, and they can indicate this to their interviewers. In spite of this, professionals do sometimes want to disclose difficult things in their family past. This has to be handled delicately, but it provides an opportunity to learn the appropriate sensitivity for dealing with similar situations when they arise while taking genograms from clients.

Interviewing a couple

This exercise gives course participants an opportunity to try out a narrative approach to marital or couple work. In the exercise, we divide people into a number of small groups, each of which will appoint two people to act as a married couple and one to act as an interviewer, while the rest are observers. The actors are given the following scenario:

> Mr and Mrs B are in their fifties. He is employed full-time and she has an afternoon job. They have two teenage children. Mrs B's father died two years ago, but the other three grandparents are alive. Mrs B often goes to her doctor with physical problems – none serious. Since Christmas, Mrs B has had panics every morning. She clings on to Mr B and cries to prevent him leaving. Mr B feels this is a medical problem and the only solution will be for his wife to take pills. Mrs B often complains to her husband that she feels little emotional support from him these days, especially since her father died, and because he has such demanding work. They have decided to come to seek help from a neutral professional about this. Discuss this for five minutes, building a few extra factors onto the story before you see the professional.

The interviewer and observers in each of the small groups then receive their own slightly different instructions:

> Mr and Mrs B are in their fifties. He is employed full-time, and she as an afternoon job. They have two teenage children. Mrs B's father died two years ago, but the other three grandparents are alive. Mrs B often sees doctors with

physical problems – none serious. Today, the couple have asked if they can see you as a neutral professional to talk about difficulties Mrs B has had since her father's death. Discuss this for 15 minutes, exploring the ideas you might have as you fetch the couple into your room.

The structure of the exercise is as follows:

- Fifteen minutes for each couple and group to sit apart and prepare.
- Thirty minutes for the interview, with the interviewer allowed to "freeze" the conversation to seek hypotheses and possible questions from the observers.
- Thirty minutes of plenary discussion concerning the pragmatic and clinical points raised.

This exercise raises a multiplicity of issues, both technical and conceptual:

1 Exercises such as this expose how little training professionals receive either in focusing simultaneously on more than one person in the family at any time, or on dealing with marital difference or conflict in particular. Course participants playing the role of interviewer here at first seem to have difficulty in eliciting the two different stories of reality that husband and wife present. They may struggle between two equally unacceptable positions. One is to treat the wife as "the real patient," implicitly siding with her husband's view of matters. The other is to treat the husband as "the real problem," consequently alienating a man who genuinely believes he has come along to help his wife get appropriate help.
2 Even though presentations such as this one must occur regularly in very many work settings in health and social care, many professionals seem ill-equipped to adopt a neutral or curious stance. They find it hard to take both points of view on board so that a couple are helped to reach an understanding of each other's somewhat incomplete story of how things got to be as they are. The exercise therefore provides an opportunity to learn the rudiments of a questioning approach where the interviewer floats non-committally between opposing positions and tries to facilitate an agreed story, rather than feeling obliged to adjudicate and then to reach a "solution" based on that adjudication.
3 Such exercises raise the question of what constitutes mental illness and what determines it. Is it legitimate, for instance, to regard Mrs B's condition as an illness when (in her view at any rate) it seems so closely connected with her family circumstances? Equally, is it fair to disqualify Mr B's view of her symptoms simply on the grounds that it is now rather unfashionable, except among some psychiatrists, to see mental symptoms in the way he does? The problem for Mr and Mrs B is not whether one of these theoretical positions will eventually prevail, but how they are to live with each other while each placing a different but acceptable construction on their experience.

4   There are also gender issues here. Mrs B's feeling that her problems are related to her personal context, and Mr B's characterisation of them as pathology, are conventionally gendered beliefs. Again, it may be tempting for people doing the exercise to choose positions based on their own gender, or their beliefs about gender. This does not necessarily mean that men will side with Mr B while women side with Mrs B. On the contrary, the kind of liberal-minded men who attend training courses in interactional skills are more likely to sympathise with Mrs B. Some of the women may ironically be impatient with her overdependence. Our task, therefore, is to facilitate a new kind of neutrality and curiosity where no value judgements are attached to beliefs and behaviour of any kind. This in turn provokes inquiries about when it is right or wrong to "adopt a position." This question itself does not have any easy answers, but it does at least open up a conversation at a more sophisticated level about the boundaries between professional and personal identities, and the difference between the interviewer's external task and moral position.

Dealing with possible child abuse

This exercise addresses a common area of difficulty that health and social care professionals encounter. The scenario, given to all participants, is as follows:

> A couple (Mr and Mrs K) are married and in their late thirties. They have a 6-week-old boy, Jeremy, their first child. A week ago, they attended the emergency department of the local hospital because Jeremy had a bruise on his leg following a fall from his changing table. The paediatricians kept the family overnight. They came to the conclusion that on the balance of probabilities, it had happened as a result of the parents' inexperience, but they had not intentionally harmed him. However, they sent a note to the family's GP suggesting she should remain alert in case of further concerns.
>
> Yesterday, Mr and Mrs K went to see their GP because Jeremy had had diarrhoea on and off for three days. The doctor felt he was not significantly ill, but the baby was listless, so she said she would prefer to ask for another paediatric assessment just to be on the safe side. The parents responded sharply and refused, saying it was impractical to spend another day and possibly night at the hospital as they had to do previously. However, they agreed to the doctor's suggestion that another practitioner could visit them at home to discuss how to cope with a new baby.

The structure of the exercise is as follows:

- Two people volunteer as Mr and Mrs K, and one as the visiting practitioner, who can choose whether to act in their normal profession (e.g. nurse, doctor, social worker) or another one if more appropriate.
- The couple go aside for 15 minutes to get into role (which may mean inventing some extra biographical details as well).
- While the couple are getting into role, the rest of the group help the practitioner to think about how to conduct this consultation.
- Twenty to thirty minutes are allowed for the consultation itself, with the practitioner being able to "freeze" the conversation for a discussion with the rest of the group.
- A plenary discussion.

The following issues usually emerge from this exercise:

1 *Safeguarding.* There is a possibility that non-accidental injury has occurred, but we cannot know if this has been tackled directly with the family or merely hinted at – as is sometimes the case. Is it a prerequisite of any sensible conversation that this now has to be brought into the open, with an inquiry as to how Mr and Mrs K experienced the imputation (or possibly undeserved exoneration)? What are the risks of pursuing this with the couple, or of not pursuing it?

2 *Ethnicity.* To make this case more complex but also more realistic and challenging, we sometimes intentionally give the family in the scenario a clear ethnic identity. It is interesting to see how participants in the exercise respond to this, with expressed or unexpressed assumptions that families of some ethnic backgrounds are more or less likely to perpetrate abuse. To those who claim that the family's name does not lead them to make assumptions of any kind, we inquire what difference it would make if their name denoted different ethnic or class identity (e.g. O'Mahoney, Patel, Cohen, Marlborough, Okolo, Wong, Abdullah) – or if the couple were younger. It is hard to resist the inference that it is impossible to practise without prejudice. The issue therefore becomes one of identifying and analysing how one's own background and that of the clients' might be influencing the interaction, and to counterbalance that by considering what alternative constructions might be put on the situation other than those one might have assumed.

3 *Relationships in the professional network.* There may be differences of view between GPs, hospital specialists, health visitors, social workers and others about the level of risk. Every time we have done this exercise, one of the thorniest difficulties centres on the couple's refusal to return to the hospital.

Although all clinical urgency has vanished, there is now a precedent for refusing recommended medical care for a baby. Although this can be read as an understandable emotional reaction to unwarranted suspicions, it may equally presage further worrying and intemperate encounters between the family and the professions. How can the professional manage such imponderables in the consultation with the family, in a way that at least minimises the risk of the worst kinds of outcomes?

Doing the exercise itself, and in conducting the discussion afterwards, we make no pretence at having definitive answers to these questions. Rather, what we hope to do is to help practitioners analyse the multiple contexts in which these cases are embedded and to learn to challenge their own unexamined assumptions. We also aim to help them to make informed decisions about practical strategies, to operationalise these strategies with thoughtful interventions based on sophisticated micro-skills, and to try to create a space for the family and the carers to create a new and more harmonious story.

Reference

Miller, L. and Halpern, H. (2012) Speed supervision. *Clinical Teacher*, 9, 14–17.

Index